MEDICAL MASTERCLASS

Rheumatology and Clinical Immunology

Disclaimer

Although every effort has been made to ensure that drug doses and other information are presented accurately in this publication, the ultimate responsibility rests with the prescribing physician. Neither the publishers nor the authors can be held responsible for any consequences arising from the use of information contained herein. Any product mentioned in this publication should be used in accordance with the prescribing information prepared by the manufacturers.

The information presented in this publication reflects the opinions of its contributors and should not be taken to represent the policy and views of the Royal College of Physicians of London, unless this is specifically stated.

Every effort has been made by the contributors to contact holders of copyright to obtain permission to reproduce copyright material. However, if any have been inadvertently overlooked, the publisher will be pleased to make the necessary arrangements at the first opportunity.

Medical Masterclass

EDITOR-IN-CHIEF

John D. Firth DM FRCP
Consultant Physician and Nephrologist
Addenbrooke's Hospital
Cambridge

Rheumatology and Clinical Immunology

EDITOR

Siraj A. Misbah MBBS MSc FRCP FRCPath
Consultant Clinical Immunologist and Honorary Senior Clinical Lecturer
Leeds General Infirmary and University of Leeds
Leeds

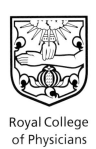

Royal College
of Physicians

Distribution Information:
Jerwood Medical Education Resource Centre
Royal College of Physicians of London
11 St. Andrews Place
Regent's Park
London NW1 4LE
United Kingdom
Tel: 0044 (0)207 935 1174 ext 422/490
Fax: 0044 (0)207 486 6653
Email: merc@rcplondon.ac.uk
Web: http://www.rcplondon.ac.uk/

Contents

List of contributors

Khalid Binymin MBChB MRCP MSc
Consultant Physician and Rheumatologist
Southport and Formby General Hospital
Southport

Hilary J. Longhurst MA MRCP PhD MRCPath
Lecturer and Honorary Senior Registrar
Department of Immunology
University of London
St. Bartholomew's Hospital, London

Siraj A. Misbah MBBS MSc FRCP FRCPath
Consultant Clinical Immunologist and
*   Honorary Senior Clinical Lecturer*
Leeds General Infirmary and University of Leeds
Leeds

Neil Snowden MB BChir MRCP MRCPath
Consultant Rheumatologist and Clinical Immunologist
North Manchester General Hospital
Manchester

Foreword

Since its foundation in 1518, the Royal College of Physicians has engaged in a wide range of activities dedicated to its overall aim of upholding and improving standards of medical practice. *Medical Masterclass* is one of the most innovative and ambitious educational resources the College has developed, and while it continues the tradition of pioneering and supporting high quality medicine, it also makes use of modern day technology by offering computer-assisted learning.

The MRCP(UK) examination is crucial to the progress of physicians through their training. Preparation is not only essential for success in the examination, but it is also important for the acquisition of requisite knowledge, skills and attitudes appropriate for further training. With a pass rate of about 40% at each sitting of the written papers, the exam is a challenge. The College wishes to encourage excellence, and with this in mind has produced *Medical Masterclass*, a comprehensive distance-learning package designed to help candidates with the preparation that is key to making the grade.

Medical Masterclass has been produced by the RCP's Education Department. It represents a formidable amount of work by Dr John Firth and his team of authors and editors. I congratulate our colleagues for this superb educational product and wholeheartedly recommend it as an invaluable MRCP(UK) study aid.

Professor Carol M. Black CBE
President of the Royal College of Physicians

Preface

Medical Masterclass comprises twelve paper-based modules, two CD-ROMs and a companion website. Its aim is to help doctors in their first few years of training to improve their medical skills and knowledge.

The twelve paper-based modules are divided as follows: two cover the scientific background to medicine, one is devoted to general clinical issues, one to emergency medicine and practical procedures, and eight cover the range of medical specialities. Medicine is often fairly straightforward when the diagnosis is clear, but patients rarely come to their doctor and say 'I've got Hodgkin's disease': they have lumps. The core material of each of the clinical specialities is defined by case presentations in the first part of each module: how do you approach the man who has lumps? Structured concise notes on specific diseases follow later. All practising doctors know that medicine is much more than knowing lots of facts about diseases: how do you tell someone they've got cancer? How do you decide when to stop treatment? Most medical texts say little about these issues: *Medical Masterclass* does not avoid them, nor does it talk in vague and abstract terms.

The two CD-ROMs each contain 30 interactive cases requiring diagnosis and treatment. The format is remarkably close to real life: you see the patient and are told the story; you have to decide how to investigate and treat; but you can't see all the results before you start to make decisions!

The companion website, which will be regularly updated, includes self-assessment questions and mock MRCP(UK) exam papers. How much do you know, and are you improving? You will see how your score compares with your previous attempts, and also how your performance compares with others who have logged on to the site.

The *Medical Masterclass* is produced by the Education Department of the Royal College of Physicians. It has been specifically designed to support candidates studying for the MRCP(UK) Examination (All Parts). I have no doubt that someone putting effort into learning through the *Medical Masterclass* would be in a strong position to impress the examiners.

John Firth
Editor-in-Chief

Acknowledgements

Medical Masterclass has been produced by a team. The names of those who have written and edited material are clearly indicated elsewhere, but without the efforts of many other people *Medical Masterclass* would not exist at all. These include Professor Lesley Rees and Mrs Winnie Wade from the Education Department of the Royal College of Physicians of London, who initiated the project; Dr Mike Stein and Dr Andy Robinson from Medschool.com and Blackwell Science respectively, who have enthusiastically supported it from the beginning; and Ms Filipa Maia and Ms Katherine Bowker, who have run the office with splendid efficiency and induced authors and editors to perform to a schedule rarely achieved. I and the whole of the team of editors and authors are immensely grateful to all of these people for the energy that they have poured into *Medical Masterclass* in various ways.

John Firth
Editor-in-Chief

x

Key features

We have created a range of icon boxes to help you identify key information and to make learning easier and more enjoyable. Here is a brief explanation:

 Clinical pointer

This icon highlights important information to be noted.

 Further information

This icon indicates the source of further information and reference.

 Hints

This icon highlights useful hints, tips and mnemonics.

Key points

This icon is used to highlight points of particular importance.

 Quote

This icon indicates useful or interesting citations from notable individuals, including well-known physicians.

 Think about

This icon indicates what the reader should reflect on after having read a passage from the text.

 Warning/Hazard

This icon is used to indicate common or important drug interactions, pitfalls of practical procedures, or when to take symptoms or signs particularly seriously.

Rheumatology and Clinical Immunology

AUTHORS:
**S.A. Misbah, N. Snowden,
H. Longhurst, K. Binymin**

EDITOR:
S.A. Misbah

EDITOR-IN-CHIEF:
J.D. Firth

1 Clinical presentations

1.1 Recurrent chest infections

Case history

A 25-year-old systems analyst is referred after three hospital admissions with pneumonia within the previous 2 years. He has had several episodes of sinusitis, recurring despite surgery, and has chronic diarrhoea. He is a non-smoker.

Clinical approach

You must decide whether this man has an underlying immunological problem and, if so, determine what it is:
• Unusually severe or frequent infections suggest the possibility of an immunodeficiency.
• Bacterial respiratory tract infections are most commonly associated with antibody deficiency, such as common variable immunodeficiency (CVID) [1].
• Primary immunodeficiencies are uncommon but are often associated with diagnostic delay of many years, with consequent avoidable morbidity and mortality [2].

History of the presenting problem

Site of infections

The respiratory tract, gut and skin are the most common sites of infection in antibody deficiency.

Identifying pathogens

Bacterial infections suggest an antibody deficiency. *Giardia* species are a common bowel pathogen. Mild CD4 deficiency may occur in CVID and manifests as recurrent herpes simplex or zoster. Any suggestion of a more severe T-cell defect should prompt you to consider a combined defect such as hyper-IgM syndrome or a 'leaky' severe combined immunodeficiency (SCID) (see Section 2.1.2, pp. 56–58).

Severity

How long do infections last? How well do they respond to antibiotics? The need for surgery or excessive time off work is an indicator of severe disease.

When did the problem start?

Common variable immunodeficiency is acquired, usually in early adulthood. If your patient has had a significant history of childhood problems, consider a late presentation of X-linked agammaglobulinaemia (XLA) (see Section 2.1.1, pp. 54–56) or a leaky SCID. Ask specifically about common childhood illnesses.

Existing medication

Is the patient taking antiepileptics—phenytoin or carbamazepine? Is he on treatment for arthritis—gold, penicillamine, sulphasalazine or methotrexate? These are reversible causes of hypogammaglobulinaemia.

Features associated with CVID

Does this man have a personal or family history of organ-specific autoimmunity? Ask about the following:
• Anaemia: pernicious anaemia and autoimmune haemolytic anaemia are common in CVID.
• Arthralgia, which is often reactive but may be septic, is caused by *Mycoplasma* spp. as well as by more conventional organisms. In CVID, granulomas may give a sarcoid-like picture.

Consequences of CVID

You need more details about this man's diarrhoea. It may simply be a result of chronic infection or bacterial overgrowth, but coeliac and inflammatory bowel disease-type enterocolitis may also occur. Ask about symptoms of bronchiectasis (see *Respiratory medicine*, Section 2.4).

Examination

General features

Assess his general appearance, growth, skin, mouth and lymph nodes, and look for hepatosplenomegaly.

The mouth is a good place to look for signs of immunodeficiency:
• Tonsils (and other lymphoid tissue) are absent in XLA
• Herpes, candidiasis or hairy oral leukoplakia is suggestive of a combined or T-cell defect
• Periodontal disease occurs in chronic granulomatous disease
• Aphthous ulcers are a non-specific sign of immunodeficiency.

Significant growth retardation is rare in CVID and suggests a long-standing, probably congenital defect. Hepato- or splenomegaly occurs in the granulomatous form of CVID, but could also be a sign of underlying lymphoproliferative disease.

Primary or secondary antibody deficiency

If this man has antibody deficiency, is it primary or secondary? In a 25 year old, once you have scrutinized his drug history, you are unlikely to find additional underlying pathology. You should, however, consider whether he may have intestinal lymphangiectasia, protein-losing enteropathy, severe nephrotic syndrome or a lymphoproliferative condition, which can cause secondary antibody deficiency.

Assess secondary damage

Look for signs of structural damage, especially bronchiectasis and rheumatological complications. Check for signs of malabsorption or vitamin deficiency.

Approach to investigations and management

Your aim is to:
• define the immunological defect
• diagnose active infections
• assess structural damage
• initiate ongoing monitoring
• give appropriate treatment.

Define the immunological defect

See Section 3.3, pp. 101–104.

Diagnose active infections

This man has several potential sites of active infection:
• Respiratory: request sputum microscopy and culture and chest radiograph if symptoms suggest active infection.
• Gastrointestinal tract: request repeated stool microscopy and culture. Do a duodenal biopsy and aspirate, looking for *Giardia* spp. and bowel changes such as villous atrophy or, rarely, lymphoid interstitial hyperplasia or lymphangiectasia. Consider colonoscopy if inflammatory bowel disease is a possibility.

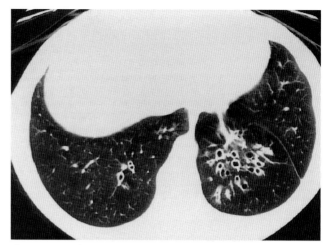

Fig. 1 CT scan showing dilated and thickened airways characteristic of bronchiectasis.

• Other sites: get samples for culture where possible. Remember that serology is likely to be unhelpful.

Assess structural damage and initiate ongoing monitoring

Get a baseline chest radiograph and computed tomography (CT) scan of the chest (Fig. 1) and sinuses. Take a radiograph of arthritic joints. Do baseline and annual lung function tests. Take blood for baseline liver function and for hepatitis B and C markers if immunoglobulin replacement is contemplated.

Give appropriate treatment

• Acute infections require a prolonged course of antibiotics.
• Long-term, severe antibody deficiencies require intravenous (or subcutaneous) immunoglobulin replacement (see Section 3.7, pp. 110–111). IgG subclass, or specific antibody deficiencies, can often be managed with prophy-lactic antibiotics, such as azithromycin 500 mg once daily for 3 days every fortnight.

Self-help

Patients with relatively rare conditions, such as CVID, are unlikely to meet others with the same condition. Put him in contact with the Primary Immunodeficiency Association (Alliance House, 12 Caxton Street, London SW1H 0QS; telephone 020 7976 7640), a self-help organization providing information and practical support [3].

Consider other causes of recurrent chest infection, many of which are associated with diarrhoea:
• Common: foreign body, HIV, ciliary dysfunction caused by smoking, cystic fibrosis.
• Uncommon: immotile cilia syndrome. Young's syndrome (obstructive azoospermia and ciliary dysfunction).

1 Spickett GP, Farrant J, North ME, Jiang-gang Z, Morgan L, Webster ADB. Common variable immunodeficiency: How many diseases? *Immunol Today* 1997; 18: 325–328.
2 Primary immunodeficiency diseases: report of an IUIS Scientific Committee. *Clin Exp Immunol* 1999; 118 (suppl 1): 1–28.
3 Primary Immunodeficiency Association: http://www.pia.org.uk.

1.2 Recurrent meningitis

Case history

A 20-year-old man is referred to your clinic after two episodes of meningococcal meningitis.

Clinical approach

Meningococcal meningitis is a serious infection with significant morbidity and mortality. Your task is to determine whether there is an underlying reason for this man's infection and, if so, to advise on action to prevent a recurrence.

Underlying causes for recurrent meningitis:
• Traumatic or congenital connection with the subarachnoid space causing a 'cerebrospinal fluid [CSF] leak'.
• Deficiency of a component of terminal pathway of complement [1] (C5, 6, 7 or 8; C9 deficiency is usually asymptomatic) or properdin or factor D in the alternative pathway (see *Immunology and immunosuppression*, Section 6).
• Other immunodeficiencies: the history will almost always reveal associated features.

• Recurrent aseptic meningitis (Mollaret's): some cases are associated with herpes simplex virus infection.
• Behçet's syndrome (see Section 2.5.5, pp. 94–95).
• Systemic lupus erythematosus (see Section 2.4.1, pp. 83–85).

History of the presenting problem

Ensure that you have enough information to confirm the diagnosis:
• Were meningococci cultured from blood or CSF?
• Were typical features of invasive meningococcal infection present?

Take this opportunity to ensure that appropriate antibiotic prophylaxis was given to your patient and his household contacts after treatment. (See *Infectious diseases*, Sections 1.14 and 1.38.)

External connection with the subarachnoid space

This is the most common cause of recurrent meningitis. It is uncommon for meningococci to cause meningitis in this setting. The causative organisms vary (*Streptococcus pneumoniae, Haemophilus influenzae*) (Fig. 2).

Ask about the following:
• Head injuries, especially fractures involving the base of the skull
• Chronic sinusitis, mastoiditis or inner-ear disease
• Previous brain or pituitary surgery.

Immunological cause

Deficiency of the terminal complement components, C5–9, and deficiencies of the alternative pathway components—properdin and factor D—are strongly associated with an

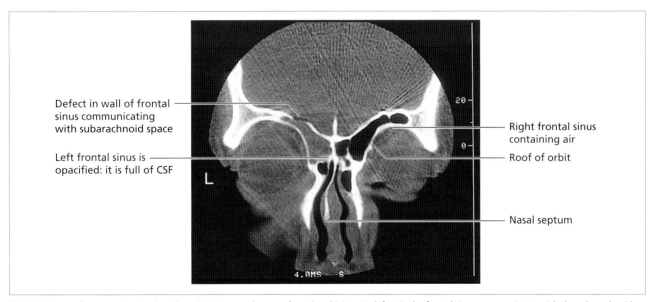

Fig. 2 CT scan of a man who developed meningitis several years after a head injury. A defect in the frontal sinus communicates with the subarachnoid space. The left frontal sinus is opacified because it is full of CSF. (With permission from Bannister BA, Begg NT, Gillespie SH. *Infectious Disease*, 2nd edn. Oxford: Blackwell Science, 2000.)

increased risk of neisserial infection and occasionally with *Escherichia coli*. Ask about gonococcal as well as meningococcal infection. Infection may be recurrent and disseminated, but is often less intense in the presence of complement deficiency.

Other immunodeficiencies are sometimes associated with recurrent meningitis. You should ask about features associated with antibody or cellular deficiencies (see Sections 2.1.1, pp. 54–56 and 2.1.2, pp. 56–58).

Family history

If the history suggests an X-linked inheritance, properdin deficiency [2] is most likely. Autosomal recessive inheritance suggests factor D or one of the terminal pathway component deficiencies.

Examination

If the patient has terminal complement or properdin deficiency, he will be asymptomatic and have no physical signs between attacks. You should look for signs of disease, previous surgery or injury that may result in a CSF leak.

Approach to investigations and management

Investigation

CSF leak

Magnetic resonance imaging (MRI) is the investigation of choice. Increase the diagnostic sensitivity by making sure that the radiologist is fully informed about the possible site and nature of the abnormality.

Complement deficiency

Fresh samples, sent on ice are required.
• Haemolytic complement assays (CH50 or CH100) measure the ability of the classic complement pathway, C1–9, to lyse red cells (Table 1).
• The AP50 (or AP100) measures lysis by the alternative pathway—factor B to complement C9.

Absence of red cell lysis implies absence of one of the factors in the assayed pathway. If either of these screening tests is abnormal, each relevant complement component should be measured individually. Occasionally, a nonfunctional complement component may be present. If no quantitative deficiency is found to account for absent lysis (and you are certain that the CH50 sample was handled correctly), you should request functional studies.

Management

Antibiotics

Prescribe long-term prophylactic phenoxymethylpenicillin 500 mg twice daily. Some organisms may, however, be resistant.

Immunization

Conjugated vaccine against *Neisseria meningitidis* type C should be given. You should also consider giving the unconjugated vaccine for types A and C in patients with a high risk of exposure. Measurements of meningococcal antibody levels can help you decide when reimmunization is necessary, although this can be unreliable. Higher levels will be required for protection in complement-deficient individuals and disease is often caused by uncommon serotypes not covered by immunization.

 Immunization will reduce, but not eliminate, the risk of recurrent meningococcal meningitis for this man. For patients with early complement component or C3 deficiency, additional immunization with Pneumovax and haemophilus conjugate vaccines is indicated.

Replacement of missing factor

This is not usually practical, because the half-life of circulating complement is extremely short. Infusions of fresh frozen (or commercially available solvent-treated) plasma would be required, with significant expense, inconvenience and some risk to your patient.

Genetic counselling

Depending on the exact deficit, the CH50 or AP50 may be used for screening of relatives.

	Classic pathway CH50	
	Normal	Abnormal
Alternative pathway AP50		
Normal	No abnormality of complement	C1–4 abnormal
Abnormal	Factor B, D or properdin abnormal	C5–9 abnormal

Table 1 Interpretation of haemolytic complement assays CH50 and AP50.

1 Fijen CA, Kuijper FJ, te Bulte MT *et al.* Assessment of complement deficiency in patients with meningococcal disease in The Netherlands. *Clin Infect Dis* 1999; 28: 98–105.
2 Linton SM, Morgan BP. Properdin deficiency and meningococcal disease—identifying those most at risk. *Clin Exp Immunol* 1999; 118: 189–191.

1.3 Recurrent facial swelling and abdominal pain

Case history

A 30-year-old housewife is referred by her dentist after an episode of facial swelling, throat tightness and abdominal pain during a dental extraction.

Clinical approach

You must differentiate C1 inhibitor deficiency from drug-induced angio-oedema and anaphylaxis. This is an important diagnosis to make—both disorders can present as medical emergencies with upper airway obstruction, but they require very different treatment and prophylaxis.

C1 inhibitor

C1 inhibitor limits activation of the early part of the classic complement cascade, as well as having a regulatory role in other inflammatory pathways. C1 inhibitor deficiency results in activation of the early components C1, -4 and -2, with release of inflammatory fragments. Other regulatory mechanisms prevent C3 breakdown or further activation of the complement pathway. (See *Immunology and immunosuppression*, Section 6.)

History of the presenting problem

Both C1 inhibitor deficiency and anaphylaxis present with facial and laryngeal oedema, but there are differences in presentation.

> In one instance, possibly in two, death resulted from a sudden oedema glottidis. (Osler, 1888 [1])

Features of C1 inhibitor deficiency

Associated abdominal pain in this woman may be the result of intestinal oedema. This strongly favours a diagnosis of C1 inhibitor deficiency and may be the presenting feature in children. Dermal swellings are common but urticaria is not associated with this condition.

Features of anaphylaxis

Urticaria, asthma and hypotension caused by generalized vasodilatation do not occur in C1 inhibitor deficiency. (See Section 2.2.1, pp. 64–66 and *Emergency medicine*, Section 1.29.)

Precipitating factors

Symptoms following trauma

Even minor trauma such as dental work can precipitate symptoms in C1 inhibitor deficiency. This can be mistaken for allergy to local anaesthetic. Ask about dermal swellings, which often follow minor knocks. Surgical procedures can precipitate catastrophic reactions, but may also have been mistaken for an allergy.

Angio-oedema precipitants

Ask about other precipitants of angio-oedema in C1 inhibitor deficiency:
• Minor infections
• Stress
• Endogenous oestrogens.

Differential diagnosis

Existing medication

Angiotensin-converting enzyme (ACE) inhibitors are a common cause of non-histamine-related angio-oedema. As symptoms do not follow immediately after taking the tablets, the patient may not link the symptoms with medication. The vast majority of people with ACE inhibitor-induced angio-oedema do not have C1 inhibitor deficiency, although it will precipitate attacks in affected people.

The following may be other drug-related causes of angio-oedema:
• Anaphylactic (IgE-induced mast cell degranulation), e.g. penicillin allergy
• Anaphylactoid (non-IgE-induced mast cell degranulation), e.g. radiographic contrast media
• Immune complex mediated, e.g. blood products.

Don't forget physical factors (cold, pressure, vibration). All of these may be associated with urticaria, which effectively excludes the diagnosis of C1 inhibitor deficiency.

Consider the aetiology

C1 inhibitor deficiency may be congenital or acquired.

Congenital

Ask about family history. Congenital C1 inhibitor deficiency is inherited in an autosomal dominant manner. Onset of symptoms is usually in adolescence. If the diagnosis is confirmed, your patient will need genetic counselling and practical advice on screening of any current or future children.

Acquired

Autoantibodies to C1 inhibitor may result in functional deficiency even if normal levels of the protein are present. These occur as a result of autoimmune (systemic lupus erythematosus [SLE], rheumatoid) or lymphoproliferative disease.

Examination

This is usually normal, unless an underlying autoimmune or lymphoproliferative disease is present.

Approach to investigations and management

Investigation

Diagnosis of C1 inhibitor deficiency

Screen for C1 inhibitor deficiency by checking serum C4 levels (Fig. 3).

 A low C4 level (with normal C3) is a hallmark of both hereditary and functional C1 inhibitor deficiency. Conversely, a normal C4 effectively excludes the diagnosis.

Associated disease

In acquired deficiency check the following:
• Blood count and film
• Immunoglobulins
• Serum and urine electrophoresis
• Antinuclear antibody (ANA)
• Rheumatoid factor
• Cryoglobulins.

Management

Acute

For severe attacks, give C1 inhibitor concentrate [2] or, if this is not available, fresh frozen plasma. Epinephrine (adrenaline) is likely to be ineffective. For mild attacks, tranexamic acid can shorten the duration.

Convalescence

For hereditary C1 inhibitor deficiency, either:
• increase production by using modified androgens such as stanozolol or danazol, or
• decrease consumption by giving tranexamic acid.

 Long-term danazol therapy may be associated with hepatocellular adenomas [3]. Monitor liver function at regular intervals and arrange annual ultrasonography of the liver.

For acquired C1 inhibitor deficiency, treat the underlying cause.

Recommend that the patient wears a Medic-Alert bracelet and alert her local accident and emergency department so that acute attacks can be appropriately treated.

ACE-induced angio-oedema

Management involves permanent withdrawal of the drug. Angiotensin II antagonists are a suitable substitute but may themselves rarely cause angio-oedema.

Anaphylaxis

See Section 2.2.1, pp. 64–66 and *Emergency medicine*, Section 1.29.

 Pregnancy and C1 inhibitor deficiency

A patient with this condition needs specific pregnancy advice:
• All androgens should be stopped before conception (to avoid risk of virilization)
• Tranexamic acid is safe after 12 weeks' gestation
• C1 inhibitor concentrate can be used for acute attacks
• Symptoms usually improve during pregnancy and specific treatment may not be required
• Prophylactic C1 inhibitor concentrate should be given for caesarean section, and may be considered for vaginal delivery.

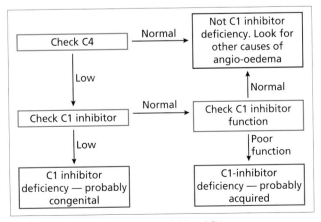

Fig. 3 Algorithm for diagnosis of C1 inhibitor deficiency.

> I find medicine worse than the malady.
> (John Fletcher 1579–1625)

Table 2 Organisms causing overwhelming infection in asplenic patients.

Bacteria	Parasites
Streptococcus pneumoniae	Malaria
Haemophilus influenzae	*Babesia* spp. (from tick bites)
Neisseria meningitides	
Staphylococcus aureus	
Klebsiella pneumoniae	
Salmonella enteriditis	
Capnocytophaga canimorsus	
(DF-2) (from dog bite)	

Surgical procedures and C1 inhibitor deficiency
- High risk: give C1 inhibitor concentrate preoperatively
- Low risk: give high-dose danazol (600 mg once daily) or stanozolol (5 mg once daily) for 6 days before and 3 days after the procedure [4]. Ensure that the C1 inhibitor concentrate is available for emergencies.

1 Osler. *Am J Med Sci* 1888; 95: 362–7.
2 Kunschak M, Engl W, Maritsch F *et al.* A randomised, controlled trial to study the efficacy and safety of C1 inhibitor concentrate in treating hereditary angioedema. *Transfusion* 1998; 38: 540–9.
3 Bork K, Pitton M, Harten P, Kock P. Hepatocellular adenomas in patients taking danazol for hereditary angioedema. *Lancet* 1999; 252: 1066–7.
4 Farkas H, Gyeney L, Gidofalvy E, Fust G, Varga L. The efficacy of short-term danazol prophylaxis in hereditary angioedema patients undergoing maxillofacial and dental procedures. *J Oral Maxillofac Surg* 1999; 57: 404–8.

1.4 Fulminant septicaemia

Case history

A 50-year-old asplenic woman presents to accident and emergency with fever and confusion. Her observations on admission confirm fever (of 39°C), tachycardia (150/min) and hypotension (blood pressure 80/40 mmHg).

Despite prompt treatment for septicaemia (see *Emergency medicine*, Sections 1.2 and 1.28, and *Infectious diseases*, Section 1.2), she develops multiorgan failure and dies. Pneumococci are subsequently isolated from her blood.

Fever in hyposplenic patients

Fever in hyposplenic patients is a medical emergency. Patients should receive parenteral penicillin before hospital admission. Do not delay in order to collect blood cultures. If your patient is already on penicillin, or you have reason to suspect a resistant organism, give ceftriaxone.

Clinical approach

The clue here is the history of splenectomy. Splenectomy predisposes to fulminant infection with encapsulated organisms and some intraerythrocytic protozoa (Table 2). The lesson is prevention: mortality of fulminant pneumococcal disease is very high but you can prevent this in many cases by offering immunization and prophylactic penicillin.

History of the presenting problem

The history, obtained from her husband, is of a flu-like illness, which started that morning. She had idiopathic thrombocytopenic purpura (ITP) 7 years ago, which required splenectomy. After this her platelet count has remained satisfactory and she has not been followed up for several years. He is unsure whether she was immunized before splenectomy.

Relevant past history

History suggestive of hyposplenism

In any patient with septicaemia, consider the possibility of hyposplenism; this does not necessarily require splenectomy and may occur with an intact spleen (functional hyposplenism).

In anyone who has had a splenectomy, ask about the following:
- Trauma
- Haematological autoimmunity
- Haematological malignancy.
  Ask about diseases associated with hyposplenism:
- Sickle cell disease
- Thalassaemia major
- Coeliac disease
- Inflammatory bowel disease.

Examination

In any patient with profound septicaemia, consider the possibility of hyposplenism. Look for:
- Splenectomy scar
- Signs of associated disorders.

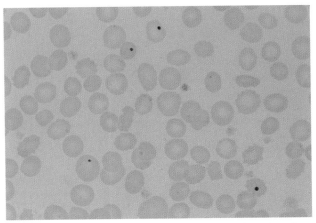

Fig. 4 Blood film depicting Howell–Jolly bodies (intraerythrocytic nuclear fragments) in a patient after splenectomy for immune thrombocytopenic purpura. (Courtesy of Dr D Swirsky, Leeds General Infirmary.)

Approach to investigations and management

Investigation

Howell–Jolly bodies on the blood film indicate hyposplenism (Fig. 4).

Management

How could this woman's death have been avoided?

Prophylaxis against infection

IMMUNIZATION

In addition to routine immunizations, you should recommend pneumococcal, *Haemophilus influenzae* type b and conjugated meningococcal C vaccines, ideally at least 2 weeks before elective splenectomy. Antibody levels will decline more quickly in hyposplenic people. Check annually after a year and expect to reimmunize after a mean of 5–10 years.

Recommend annual influenza vaccine, because influenza confers a high risk of secondary bacterial infection. Additional vaccines, such as meningococcus A and C, may be used in situations of high risk, such as travel to an endemic area.

 Penicillin should be continued even if levels of pneumococcal antibodies are high. Commercially available pneumococcal vaccines contain only 23 serotypes of pneumococci of varying immunogenicity; high antibody levels to some serotypes may mask inadequate levels of antibody to others.

ANTIMICROBIAL PROPHYLAXIS

Prescribe life-long penicillin and give your patients a supply of amoxycillin to enable early initiation of treatment if they develop a fever. Ensure that they receive antimalarials if travelling to a high-risk area.

OTHER PRECAUTIONS

Animal and tick bites can be dangerous. Clean the wound and consider a short course of antibiotics.

Advise your patient to wear a Medic-Alert bracelet.

 Be careful with antibiotic prophylaxis. Recommendations may need to be modified to accommodate your patient.
- Is she or he allergic to penicillin?
- Does she or he live in an area with a high prevalence of penicillin-resistant pneumococci?

Local microbiologists will be able to help here.

 Working party of the British Committee for Standards in Haematology Clinical Haematology Task Force. Guidelines for the prevention and treatment of infection in patients with an absent or dysfunctional spleen. *BMJ* 1996; 312: 430–434.

1.5 Recurrent skin abscesses

Case study

A 15-year-old boy is referred for investigation of recurrent skin abscesses.

Clinical approach

Recurrent skin abscesses are common. They are distressing, expensive in time and resources, but are not usually associated with underlying immunodeficiency. However, they may occasionally be the presenting feature of a life-threatening condition such as chronic granulomatous disease (CGD) (Table 3). You must be sure not to miss the occasional serious immunodeficiency, while providing practical advice for controlling the problem to those in whom this diagnosis is excluded.

Table 3 Differential diagnosis of recurrent skin abscesses.

Common	Rare
Staphylococcal colonization	Chronic granulomatous disease (CGD)
	Neutrophil G6PD deficiency
	Neutrophil myeloperoxidase deficiency
	Antibody deficiency
	Hyper-IgE (Job's) syndrome
	Wiskott–Aldrich syndrome
	Combined deficiencies

G6PD, glucose-6-phosphate dehydrogenase.

Chronic granulomatous disease

Phagocytes of patients with CGD [1] cannot efficiently kill organisms that they have engulfed, leading to granuloma or abscess formation and failure to clear the infection.

History of the presenting problem

Types of abscesses

Ask about the abscesses:
- Are they large boils, needing surgical drainage, or smaller pustules?
- When did they start?
- How frequently do they occur?

A history of problems going back to childhood or infancy makes a congenital problem more likely.

Does each abscess respond rapidly to conventional treatment? This makes immunodeficiency less likely.

Risk of staphylococcal skin colonization

Ask about chronic skin conditions, particularly eczema. Does the patient have diabetes?

Severe eczema causes damage to the protective barrier of the skin and is associated with staphylococcal colonization. It is also a feature of two primary immunodeficiencies. Both are very rare, especially in adults.

Hyper-IgE (Job's) syndrome [1]

Severe infections, especially skin and chest with pneumatoceles, failure to lose primary dentition, abnormal facies and grossly elevated serum IgE (this is not specific for the hyper-IgE syndrome because many patients with atopic eczema have comparable IgE levels).

Wiskott–Aldrich syndrome [2]

X-linked combined (cellular and antibody) immunodeficiency, with severe infections. Thrombocytopenia with abnormally small platelets on the blood film.

Features of immunodeficiency

Ask about the following:
- Has there been associated invasive disease, abscesses of internal organs, chronic periodontitis or persistent lymphadenopathy?
- Did he have any problems with his BCG immunization?
- Are there features of other immunodeficiencies? (see Section 3.3, pp. 101–104.)
- Has he been infected with unusual organisms? Review notes and microbiology reports looking for evidence of *Aspergillus*, *Klebsiella*, *Serratia*, *Burkholderia* spp., as well as

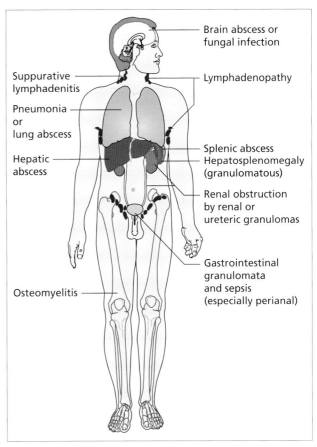

Fig. 5 Common sites of pathology in chronic granulomatous disease (CGD).

the more commonplace *Staphylococcus* spp., *E. coli* and *Salmonella* spp.

Recurrent infections with catalase-positive bacteria and *Aspergillus* spp. are characteristic of serious neutrophil defects such as CGD (Fig. 5).

Family history

Have there been any premature deaths in the family, or unusual infections? CGD is X-linked in 65% of cases, the rest being autosomal recessive.

Abscesses resulting from staphylococcal colonization often affect several members of the household—ask about flatmates and girlfriends as well as blood relatives.

Examination

Skin

Look at his skin:
- Is it eczematous?
- Are there excoriations that could be possible sites of entry for pathogens?
- Have the abscesses healed well, or are there scars suggestive of deep and severe infections?

General

Look in his mouth. Ulcers and gum disease are common with neutrophil defects. Does he have signs of chronic lung disease, lymphadenopathy or hepatosplenomegaly? These are common in CGD.

Approach to investigations and management

 Nature has provided ... in the phagocytes ... a natural means of ... destroying all disease germs. There is at bottom only one genuine scientific treatment for all diseases, and that is to stimulate the phagocytes ... drugs are a delusion. (George Bernard Shaw, from *The Doctor's Dilemma*, 1913)

Investigation

Check his blood count, immunoglobulins and glucose. Take samples from abscesses, looking for unusual organisms. Take swabs from the hairline, nose and perineum, looking for *Staphylococcus aureus*.

Exclude CGD

The nitroblue tetrazolium (NBT) slide test assesses the integrity of the neutrophil respiratory burst (NADPH oxidase system). In neutrophil killing defects (CGD, neutrophil glucose-6-phosphate dehydrogenase [G6PD] or myeloperoxidase deficiency), neutrophils fail to reduce the NBT crystals that they have phagocytosed (Fig. 6).

Cytometric measurement by fluorescent flow of the neutrophil respiratory burst is more sensitive but not universally available.

If the NBT screening test suggests a defect, do the following:
- Check for the absence of individual NADPH subunits
- If the NADPH system is intact, consider G6PD and myeloperoxidase deficiency as alternative causes for the defective NBT test.

Management

No immunological cause is found

Treat eczema (see *Dermatology*, Sections 2.7 and 2.8) and optimize control of diabetes (see *Endocrinology*, Section 2.6). Reduce staphylococcal skin colonization:
- Bath or shower daily using an antiseptic preparation such as povidone–iodine all over the body, including the hair.
- Each person should use his or her own towel, which should be changed every day.
- Consider a short course (>10 days) of a topical antibiotic, such as Naseptin or, in resistant cases, mupirocin to the nasal vestibule.

At least 2 weeks' treatment, and often considerably longer, is required.

In cases of staphylococcal carriage, every member of the patient's household should be treated because recolonization from untreated people will occur.

Chronic granulomatous disease

Prescribe prophylactic antibiotics (co-trimoxazole) and antifungal therapy (itraconazole). Consider interferon-γ prophylaxis or bone marrow transplant in difficult cases.

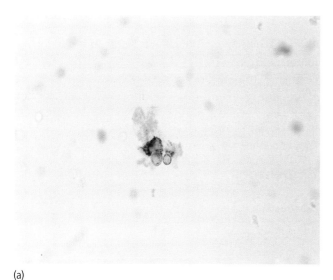
(a)

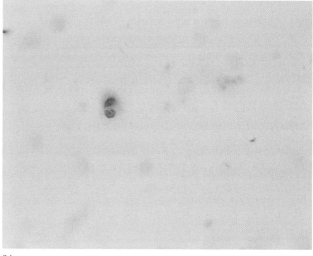
(b)

Fig. 6 The nitroblue tetrazolium (NBT) test: activated neutrophils are tested for their ability to phagocytose and reduce NBT. (a) Reduced NBT is seen as dark-blue crystals. (b) Unstimulated neutrophils, or stimulated neutrophils from patients who have CGD fail to reduce NBT. Blood from carriers of CGD contain a mixture of normal and abnormal neutrophils.

Table 4 Prevention of infection in chronic granulomatous disease.

Problem	Intervention
Avoid bacterial infection	Keep immunizations up to date
	Clean all cuts immediately and rinse with antiseptic or hydrogen peroxide (1.5% solution)
	Use hydrogen peroxide mouthwash after toothbrushing to reduce gingivitis
	Antibiotic prophylaxis is necessary for dental work
Avoid fungal spores	Avoid hay, wood chips and grass clippings
	Do not enter barns or caves
	Do not repot houseplants
	For cut flowers, use a teaspoon of bleach in the water
	Avoid newly constructed or renovated buildings until they have been thoroughly cleaned
General	Do not smoke

You should give this boy detailed instructions on the personal precautions he should take to avoid infection (Table 4).

Acute infections—see Section 2.1.3, pp. 59–60.

GENETIC COUNSELLING

Carriers of CGD can be identified by the NBT test (see Fig. 6) and by molecular analysis. Prenatal diagnosis is possible. Molecular characterization of the defect is important for genetic counselling of this boy and his family, especially if the mode of inheritance is not clear from the family history.

1 CGD Association Inc., 2616 Monterey Road, San Marino, CA 91108–1646, USA.
2 CGD Research Trust/Support Group. Seafields, Shootersway Lane, Berkhamstead, Herts HP4 3NP, UK.
3 Segal AW. The NADP oxidase and chronic granulomatous disease. *Mol Med Today* 1996; 2: 129–35.
4 Grimbacher B, Holland SM, Gallin JI *et al*. Hyper-IgE syndrome with recurrent infections—an autosomal dominant multisystem disorder. *N Engl J Med* 1999; 340: 692–701.
5 Thrasher AJ, Kinnon C. Minireview: The Wiskott–Aldrich syndrome. *Clin Exp Immunol* 2000; 120: 1–9.

1.6 Chronic atypical mycobacterial infection

Case history

Respiratory physicians refer a 21-year-old student who has mycobacterial disease of his skin, lungs, lymph nodes and liver. Biopsies show granulomas with acid-fast bacilli. Cultures grow *Mycobacterium avium-intracellulare* (MAI) complex. Investigations for HIV are negative. Despite treatment, he is getting worse.

Clinical approach

Extreme susceptibility to mycobacterial disease in the absence of obvious immunodeficiency is suggestive of defects of interferon-γ receptors (IFNγR) or interleukin-12 (IL12) and its receptor (IL12R) (see Fig. 32, p. 61) [1]. You must confirm this diagnosis and suggest appropriate treatment.

History of the presenting problem

Mycobacterial disease

This should include details of site of infection and response to treatment. Disseminated or difficult-to-treat disease is characteristic. Has he had BCG immunization? Was there disseminated disease? Was healing significantly delayed?

Salmonella Infection

Some types of IFNγR/IL12/IL12R defect are associated with susceptibility to intracellular bacterial infections, particularly *Salmonella* spp.

Other immunodeficiencies

Defects of IFNγR, IL12 and IL12R are extremely rare. Remember to consider other diagnoses, particularly combined defects or HIV, which may present with disseminated MAI infection.

Family history

Defects of IFNγR, IL12 and IL12R are a heterogeneous group but most are inherited in either an autosomal dominant or an autosomal recessive manner. Genetic counselling and advice on prophylaxis to affected family members are important. They should avoid BCG and limit their exposure to environmental mycobacteria by boiling drinking water.

Examination

A general examination is required. The aim is to:
• document the extent of disease—this is essential in monitoring the response to treatment
• exclude other immunodeficiencies.

Approach to investigations and management

Documentation of the exact defect is rarely necessary for treatment but may help in determining the prognosis.

Defining the defect

Arrange with the laboratory to assay IFNγ and IL12 secretion by stimulated lymphocytes. Low levels of these cytokines will occur in any IFNγR/IL12/IL12R deficiency. In defects of IFNγR, macrophages fail to respond to IFNγ stimulation. Defining the exact defect is not a routine assay but several research groups would be able to undertake this.

Other investigations

• Blood count: pancytopenia is associated with chronic mycobacterial disease.
• Renal and liver function may be impaired as a result of direct effects of mycobacterial invasion, granulomas or the effects of antimycobacterial drugs.
• Immunoglobulins are usually raised.
• Lymphocyte subsets: there may be a lymphopenia. In particular, some patients have a CD4 lymphopenia which may occasionally be associated with opportunistic infection such as pneumocystis pneumonia.
• Lymphocyte proliferation may be normal when stimulated by PHA (phytohaemagglutinin), but responses to PPD (purified protein derivative) vary.

Management

Once an IFNγR/IL12/IL12R defect is confirmed, a therapeutic trial of therapeutic IFNγ is justified [2].

The usual dose is 25–50 µg three times per week, and prolonged treatment for months or years is required. You should continue antimycobacterial treatment.

1 Jouanguy E, Döffinger R, Dupuis S *et al.* IL-12 and IFN-γ in host defence against mycobacteria and salmonella in mice and men. *Curr Opin Immunol* 1999; 11: 346–351.
2 Holland S, Eisenstein E, Kuhns D *et al.* Treatment of refractory disseminated non-tuberculous mycobacterial infection with interferon gamma. *N Engl J Med* 1994; 330: 1348–1355.

1.7 Collapse during a restaurant meal

Case history

A 19-year-old medical student is admitted with facial swelling, difficulty in breathing and a generalized urticarial rash. Symptoms began minutes after starting her meal in a local restaurant.

Clinical approach

This is a medical emergency. Your patient has typical features of anaphylaxis and, without prompt treatment, she may die from respiratory tract obstruction, bronchoconstriction or hypotension. If the patient looks as though she is about to arrest, then call the cardiac resuscitation team immediately—do not wait for the woman's heart to stop! If they are not so severely ill, proceed as follows:
1 *Brief* assessment
2 Resuscitation
3 History
4 Examination
5 Investigations.

Brief assessment

When the patient is *in extremis* you should take no more than a few seconds for a brief assessment. Look for features of anaphylaxis.

Upper and lower airway obstruction

Note the following:
• Can the patient speak?
• Can she swallow?
• Look in her mouth—note degree of facial, tongue and laryngeal swelling.
• Stridor or wheeze—absence of these may indicate very poor air entry and incipient respiratory arrest.
• Increased respiratory rate, indrawing of intercostals, chest expansion.

Table 5 Differential diagnosis of facial and laryngeal swelling.

Common	Allergy, including anaphylaxis Anaphylactoid reactions (usually to drugs) Salicylate hypersensitivity Infection: erysipelas, dental infections, parotitis, quinsy Trauma, including burns.
Must consider	C1 inhibitor deficiency

Vasodilatation

Is she inappropriately vasodilated? Look for erythema. Check the blood pressure.

Other features

Does she have urticaria, rhinitis, vomiting or diarrhoea? Does she have a Medic-Alert bracelet?

Your initial assessment should allow you to distinguish anaphylaxis from other common causes of laryngeal swelling (Table 5), but C1 inhibitor deficiency should not be forgotten, especially if the response to epinephrine is poor (see Section 1.3, pp. 7–8).

Consider panic attacks. These may cause dramatic breathlessness, with loud upper airway noises and occasionally erythema, but other features are absent.

Definition of anaphylaxis

One or more of the following:
- Laryngeal oedema
- Bronchoconstriction
- Hypotension.

It is caused by IgE-mediated mast cell degranulation. Abdominal cramps with severe vomiting and diarrhoea may occur. Anaphylactoid reactions are caused by non-IgE-mediated mast cell degranulation but are otherwise identical.

Resuscitation

While you are conducting the assessment, give high-flow oxygen and get emergency drugs prepared. If airway obstruction is the dominant problem, the patient will be most comfortable sitting; if hypotension, then lying flat. Then:

1 Give epinephrine 0.5 mg (0.5 mL of 1 : 1000) intramuscularly [1]. Most patients with anaphylaxis or anaphylactoid reactions respond promptly to this treatment, but repeat after 5 min if there is no response or if symptoms recur.

2 Establish intravenous access, and if the patient is hypotensive give 1–2 L of physiological (0.9%) saline.

3 Give an antihistamine, such as chlorpheniramine 10–20 mg, and hydrocortisone 100–500 mg (each by intramuscular or slow intravenous injection) to help minimize later reactions.

4 Recheck the patient's BP and listen to her chest—a salbutamol nebulizer will help any residual bronchoconstriction, and intravenous salbutamol may be necessary if the patient has recently taken a β blocker.

History of the presenting problem

In all cases of possible anaphylaxis, the history is crucial. Anaphylactic reactions usually occur within minutes of encountering the allergen. Life-threatening reactions virtually never occur more than 30 min after contact.

What did she eat?

You will need a list of all the ingredients from her meal. Get her friends to contact the chef as soon as possible.

Hidden allergens

Nuts, nut oils and spices are very common allergens that may be overlooked. Contact with latex and insect stings is unlikely to apply here, but should be considered in other cases.

Previous episodes

Have there been previous episodes, perhaps less severe? Does she have any known allergies? Atopic people (with eczema, asthma or hayfever) have a greater risk of anaphylaxis. A history of heart disease or hypertension will increase the risks of epinephrine treatment.

Drug history

The following drugs make treatment of anaphylaxis difficult or dangerous and should be avoided in future:
- β Blockers will inhibit the response to epinephrine
- Tricyclic antidepressants, monoamine oxidase inhibitors and cocaine potentiate epinephrine.

Approach to investigations and management

Investigations

- Serum mast cell tryptase: samples should be taken within 6 h. Raised levels will confirm the anaphylactic/anaphylactoid nature of the reaction. This is invaluable if the diagnosis is later questioned.
- Specific IgE for suspect allergens: radioallergosorbent 'RAST' or 'CAP' tests may occasionally be negative

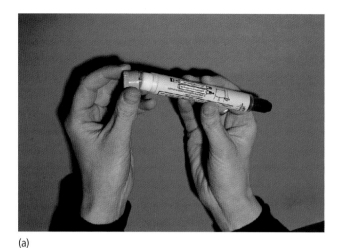
(a)

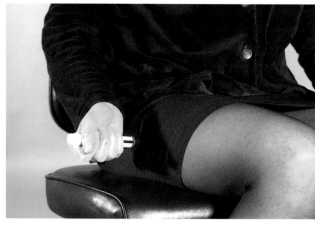
(b)

Fig. 7 Use of EpiPen: (a) take cap off back of EpiPen. (b) Holding the pen as shown, press firmly to the lateral part of the thigh, through clothes if necessary. A click will be felt as the epinephrine is injected. Hold for 10 s. After epinephrine self-administration, patients should seek urgent medical attention, because benefit may be temporary. A second 'back-up' epinephrine dose should be provided for use if symptoms do not improve or recur en route to hospital.

immediately after an episode of anaphylaxis. If in doubt, repeat at a later date.

Observation

The patient should be kept under observation for at least 12 h: biphasic anaphylactic reactions occasionally occur.

Advice to your patient

Avoidance

She must avoid any potential allergens. The advice of a dietitian is helpful for allergens such as nuts, which may be hidden ingredients.

Epinephrine

For anyone who has had a life-threatening reaction, epinephrine for self-administration should normally be prescribed. Simply giving them an epinephrine Min-I-Jet or EpiPen (Fig. 7) is not enough; it is essential for patients to receive appropriate training and education in when and how to inject themselves.

Further assessment

Refer your patient to the allergy clinic, where they will perform skinprick testing or measure specific IgE to candidate allergens. The history is vital for proper choice and interpretation of these tests; false positives and negatives are common (see Sections 2.2.1, pp. 64–66 and 2.2.3, pp. 67–68). In people with asthma, ensure that asthmatic control is optimal.

Asthma and food allergy

In patients with food allergy, poorly controlled asthma is an important risk factor for fatal anaphylaxis, underlining the need for optimal asthma control in these patients.

See *Emergency medicine*, Section 1.29.
1 Project Team of the Resuscitation Council (UK). Emergency treatment of anaphylactic reactions. *J Accid Emerg Med* 1999; 16: 243–247.

1.8 Flushing and skin rash

Case history

A 45-year-old woman presents with a 3-year history of episodic facial flushing and an urticarial rash.

Clinical approach

There are many causes of flushing, but the simultaneous occurrence of flushing and urticaria points to mast cell overactivity.

Flushing in a 45-year-old woman raises the question of a wide spectrum of disorders ranging from an early menopause to disorders caused by release of endogenous vasoactive mediators (Table 6). In this case, where there is both flushing and urticaria, you need to consider whether her symptoms are triggered by underlying allergy or reflect systemic mastocytosis [1].

Table 6 Differential diagnosis of flushing.

Disorder	Comments and key investigations
Physiological/idiopathic	Confined to exposed skin, e.g. face, neck Sometimes associated with palpitations, syncope No biochemical abnormality
Menopause	Woman >45 years with menstrual irregularities Males after orchidectomy Gonadotrophin levels are unreliable markers of the perimenopause
Carcinoid	Often postprandial flushing associated with diarrhoea and/or wheeze ↑ 24-h urinary 5-HIAA
Medullary carcinoma of the thyroid	Either sporadic or associated with multiple endocrine neoplasia syndromes ↑ Serum calcitonin
Mastocytosis	Flushing associated with urticaria, pruritis and/or diarrhoea Mast cell infiltration on skin/bone marrow biopsy ↑ Plasma tryptase, ↑ urinary methylhistamine
Drugs	Antidepressants, metronidazole (with alcohol), nicotinic acid

5-HIAA, 5-hydroxyindole acetic acid.

History of the presenting problem

Allergy or systemic mastocytosis

The history is crucial in establishing an allergic trigger. A consistent link with foods or drugs or background atopy should suggest possible allergy. Ask about the following:
• Frequency of symptoms: completely asymptomatic phases between episodes may occur with either allergy or systemic mastocytosis, although the most common rash of systemic mastocytosis—urticaria pigmentosa—tends to be fixed.
• Itching: does scratching or mild trauma cause more urticarial lesions to appear (Darier's sign)? This is a characteristic feature of urticaria pigmentosa.

Associated symptoms

Ask about the following:
• Gastrointestinal symptoms: diarrhoea, abdominal pain. Symptomatic peptic ulcers occur in 50% of patients with systemic mastocytosis.
• Palpitations.
• Constitutional symptoms: prolonged fatigue.

Examination

General

Concentrate on the skin:
• Note distribution of urticaria
• Look for cutaneous features of mastocytosis
• Look for Darier's sign
• Look for hepatosplenomegaly and lymphadenopathy caused by mast cell infiltration.

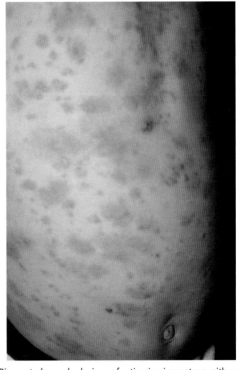

Fig. 8 Pigmented macular lesions of urticaria pigmentosa with urtication. (Courtesy of Dr M Goodfield, Leeds General Infirmary.)

Urticaria pigmentosa is characterized by a maculo-papular rash with plaques (Fig. 8).

Approach to investigations and management

Investigations

• Allergy: if the history suggests an allergic trigger, perform appropriate skinprick tests and check allergen-specific IgE.

• Mastocytosis: you need to demonstrate mast cell over-activity both histologically and biochemically.

> Histological demonstration of mast cell hyperplasia in skin and/or bone marrow, combined with biochemical evidence of elevated mast cell mediators (plasma tryptase, urinary methylhistamine), is required to establish a diagnosis of systemic mastocytosis. Measurements of mast cell mediators may be normal in mastocytosis confined to the skin.

Management

• Confirmed allergy: avoid exposure to offending allergen and symptomatic antihistamines.
• Confirmed mastocytosis: mainstay of management is histamine blockade using a combination of H_1- and H_2-receptor blockers [2] to control cutaneous symptoms and gastric acid production, respectively.

> Beware risk of severe adverse reactions with opiate analgesia and general anaesthesia.

> See *Endocrinology*, Section 1.15.
> 1 Golkar L, Bernhard JD. Mastocytosis [seminar]. *Lancet* 1997; 349: 1379–1385.
> 2 Pauls JD, Brems J, Pockros PJ *et al.* Mastocytosis—diverse presentations and outcomes. *Arch Intern Med* 1999; 159: 401–405.

1.9 Drug-induced anaphylaxis

Case histories

Case A

A 52-year-old woman is referred to an allergy clinic with a suspected food allergy. Three weeks earlier she had been admitted with a generalized rash, bronchospasm, facial swelling and a blood pressure of 70/50 mmHg. She had become unwell shortly after eating a meal of home-made chicken curry and a banana, all foods that she had eaten previously without problems. The day before she became unwell she had visited her general practitioner because of back pain and received a prescription for diclofenac. She had taken the first tablet with the meal described above. On questioning, she did not have any history of atopy, but she reported previous transient episodes of an urticarial rash over the last 6 months, associated with swelling of her upper lip on one occasion. She had attributed her episode of anaphylaxis to bananas, and since then had avoided this and all other fruit.

Case B

A 55-year-old woman visited her general practitioner with symptoms suggestive of a urinary tract infection and received a prescription for co-amoxiclav. She had no known history of drug allergy and her only past medical history was of hypertension treated with propranolol. Within minutes of taking the first antibiotic tablet she developed wheezing and dizziness, and an ambulance was called. On admission to hospital, she was cyanosed and in severe respiratory distress. A sparse urticarial rash was present on her trunk.

Clinical approach

In principle, nothing could be simpler than prevention of further attacks of drug-induced anaphylaxis: one merely has to identify the offending drug and avoid it. In practice, management is complicated by the following:
• Difficulty identifying the triggering drug, particularly where multiple drugs are used before the adverse reaction.
• The pathophysiology of the adverse reaction. These can be classic IgE-mediated type I hypersensitivity reactions, or non-IgE-mediated mast cell degranulation, as the patient in case A. In this patient, a non-steroidal anti-inflammatory drug (NSAID) has triggered severe mast cell degranulation in a patient with pre-existing mild chronic urticaria and angio-oedema [1].
• The pattern of cross-reactivity between different drugs, e.g. type I hypersensitivity to penicillins, will often be associated with the potential for similar reactions to cephalosporins [2].

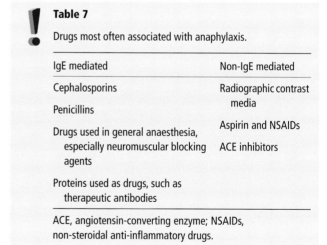

Table 7

Drugs most often associated with anaphylaxis.

IgE mediated	Non-IgE mediated
Cephalosporins	Radiographic contrast media
Penicillins	
Drugs used in general anaesthesia, especially neuromuscular blocking agents	Aspirin and NSAIDs
	ACE inhibitors
Proteins used as drugs, such as therapeutic antibodies	
ACE, angiotensin-converting enzyme; NSAIDs, non-steroidal anti-inflammatory drugs.	

History of the presenting problem

> The history is the main diagnostic tool in the assessment of drug allergy. A painstaking history is therefore essential.

Particular attention should be given to the following:
• The events immediately preceding and during the reaction. This may need to be obtained from witnesses if the patient's consciousness was impaired. Does the history suggest anaphylaxis or some cause of collapse such as a simple faint, cardiac syncope or epilepsy (see *Emergency medicine*, Section 1.6 and *Cardiology*, Sections 1.2 and 1.3). Not all the components of a full-blown anaphylactic reaction need be present for a diagnosis to be made—isolated bronchospasm or severe angio-oedema are just as important to identify.
• Previous use of any drugs: drugs taken without problems in the recent past are unlikely to be the cause.
• Previous reactions to any drugs.
• Need this be drug induced? Could the reaction be triggered by other environmental allergens, e.g. latex?
• Use of drugs that may trigger anaphylaxis, urticaria or angio-oedema by non-immunological means, such as NSAIDs or ACE inhibitors.
• Use of drugs that may worsen an anaphylactic reaction, especially β blockers.
• Presence of conditions that may increase the hazards of severe mast cell degranulation, such as unstable asthma or ischaemic heart disease.

Examination

See Section 1.7 (pp. 14–16) for details of the examination of a patient with anaphylaxis. At the time of assessment in the outpatient clinic, examination is invariably normal.

> ! The patient who gives a history of reactions to multiple drugs presents particular difficulties. Multiple drug allergies are extremely rare. Most patients who report multiple reactions have either:
> • idiopathic urticaria and angio-oedema—reactions can be precipitated by some drugs (such as NSAIDs), but also occur spontaneously (when they are often wrongly attributed to outside events); or
> • a somatization disorder—physiological changes caused by stress are perceived as being triggered by external events.

Investigations and management

Investigation

These are of limited utility [3]. If there is uncertainty regarding the cause of an episode of collapse, then serial measurements of serum mast cell tryptase may be useful.

Investigations to identify the triggering allergen include skin prick testing and measurement of specific IgE in serum. These can be used only for IgE-dependent reactions and even then are useful only in a small proportion of cases. Skin testing is difficult because the triggering allergen is often a subtle chemical modification of the administered drug, and use of simple solutions of the drug is likely to lead to false-negative results. Skin tests are of most use in the assessment of anaphylaxis associated with β-lactam antibiotics and general anaesthetic drugs. In the latter case, they can be used to pinpoint the likely allergen out of a cocktail of administered drugs.

Management

The cornerstone of management is avoidance of the suspected drug. Management of acute anaphylactic reactions is described in Sections 1.7, pp. 14–16 and 2.2.1, pp. 64–66.

> • The drug(s) to be avoided should be clearly recorded on the front of the patient's case notes.
> • The patient should be encouraged to wear a Medic-Alert (or equivalent) necklace or bracelet giving details of the allergy.

> See *Clinical pharmacology*, Section 4.
> 1 Stevenson DD. Adverse reactions to non-steroidal anti-inflammatory drugs. *Immunol Allergy Clin* 1998; 18: 773–798.
> 2 Mendelson LM. Adverse reactions to β-lactam antibiotics. *Immunol Allergy Clin* 1998; 18: 745–758.
> 3 Weiss ME, Adkinson NF. Diagnostic testing for drug hypersensitivity. *Immunol Allergy Clin* 1998; 18: 731–744.

1.10 Arthralgia, purpuric rash and renal impairment

Case history

A 50-year-old woman presents with a 2-year history of joint pains and a purpuric rash. Initial investigations reveal a negative antinuclear antibody (ANA) and renal impairment.

Clinical approach

The differential diagnoses for this constellation of clinical problems encompass lupus and the systemic vasculitides (Table 8). Lupus is effectively excluded by the negative ANA. Of the vasculitides, type II mixed cryoglobulinaemia [1] would fit her clinical problems well and should be considered a prime working diagnosis. Other small vessel vasculitides such as Wegener's granulomatosis and microscopic polyangiitis (MPA) (see Section 2.5, pp. 88–96) may also present in this manner, but the long history would be unusual.

Table 8 Differential diagnosis of arthralgia, purpuric rash and renal impairment.

Disorder	Key investigation
Lupus	Antinuclear antibody
Mixed cryoglobulinaemia	Cryoglobulins, C3, C4, rheumatoid factor
Wegener's granulomatosis and microscopic polyangiitis	ANCA, tissue biopsy
Rheumatoid vasculitis	Clinically apparent because it develops on a background of severe rheumatoid disease
Henoch–Schönlein purpura	Rare in this age group and with such a long history
	Tissue biopsy (skin, kidney) showing IgA deposition would make the diagnosis

History of the presenting problem

Cryoglobulinaemia

Is cryoglobulinaemia the explanation? Symptoms in mixed cryoglobulinaemia are the result of a combination of immune complex-induced vasculitis and vascular obstruction by cryoglobulin [2]. Your questions should therefore focus on those organs likely to be affected by systemic vasculitis, i.e. skin, joints, kidneys.

Skin

What is the nature of the rash?
• A purpuric rash affecting the lower limbs is present in >90% of patients with mixed cryoglobulinaemia (Fig. 9).
• Ask about leg ulcers, which are a feature of severe cutaneous vasculitis.

Has there been poor circulation in the hands, feet and nose?
• Ask about Raynaud's phenomenon.

Joints

What is the nature of the joint pain? Ask about the following:
• Onset and course of pain
• Distribution and symmetry: symmetrical arthralgia affecting the hands, knees, ankles and elbows is common in mixed cryoglobulinaemia, but rarely progresses to frank arthritis.

Kidneys

What is the renal involvement? Glomerulonephritis occurs in about 50% of cases of mixed cryoglobulinaemia (Fig. 9) but remains asymptomatic in the early stages.

With established renal disease, oedema and hypertension are common manifestations.

Alternative diagnosis

Are there features to suggest one of the alternative diagnoses listed in Table 8?
• Ask directly about problems with the nose (bleeding, discharge) and ears (deafness, discharge), which would suggest Wegener's granulomatosis.
• Is there anything to support the diagnosis of lupus, e.g. pleurisy, pericarditis, photosensitive rash (see Section 1.11, pp. 22–24).

Relevant past history

Previous history may be unhelpful but ask about Sjögren's syndrome, lupus and rheumatoid arthritis because cryoglobulinaemic vasculitis can occur as a complication of any of these disorders.

 Enquire about exposure to blood products because hepatitis C virus infection (HCV) now accounts for >70% of cases of mixed cryoglobulinaemia.

Examination

• General: note type and distribution of rash, and look for leg ulcers, pallor and oedema. Check blood pressure—hypertension may occur secondary to renal disease.
• Joints: look for evidence of synovitis—are the joints painful with limited movement?
• Neurological: examination is required only if the history suggests mononeuritis multiplex.

Approach to investigations and management

Investigations

Immunological tests

CRYOGLOBULINS

The key to detecting cryoglobulins is meticulous attention to detail. Collect a clotted sample of blood at 37°C and transport immediately to the immunology laboratory. Once a cryoglobulin has been detected (see Fig. 9), it is essential to characterize the type in view of the different disease associations (Table 9).

SERUM COMPLEMENT C3 AND C4

Like any immune complex, mixed cryoglobulins activate the classic complement pathway.

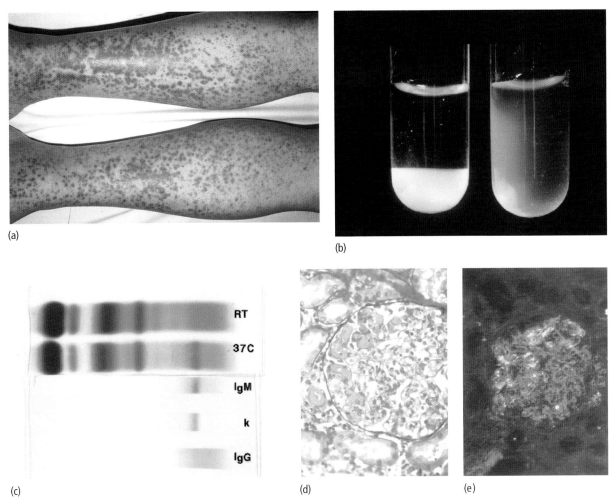

Fig. 9 Clinical and laboratory manifestations of mixed cryoglobulinaemia in a patient with hepatitis C. (a) Palpable purpura caused by cutaneous vasculitis. (b) Stored serum showing cryoprecipitate after 24 h incubation at 4°C (left), and redissolving on heating to 37°C (right). (c) Zone electrophoresis of serum collected at 37°C shows the redissolved cryoprecipitate as a discrete band in the gamma region, which on immunofixation is shown to be composed of monoclonal IgM κ and polyclonal IgG. Note the absence of γ band in sample collected at room temperature (RT). (d) Renal biopsy showing eosinophilic glomerular deposits of cryoglobulin (pseudothrombi), corresponding to IgG deposits (e) on immunofluorescence. (With permission from Graham A. *Arthritis Rheum* 1992; 35: 1107.)

Table 9 Classification of cryoglobulins.

Type	Composition	Disease associations
I	Composed entirely of monoclonal immunoglobulin, usually IgM or IgG	Waldenström's macroglobulinaemia Myeloma Lymphoproliferative disease
II	Monoclonal IgM rheumatoid factor plus polyclonal IgG	Infections, particularly hepatitis C Autoimmune Lupus Sjögren's syndrome Rheumatoid arthritis A minority of cases are labelled 'idiopathic' (mixed essential cryoglobulinaemia)
III	Polyclonal IgM rheumatoid factor plus polyclonal IgG	

Types II and III cryoglobulins have overlapping disease associations.

 A markedly low C4 occurs in >90% of patients with mixed cryoglobulinaemia, as a result of classic pathway activation.

RHEUMATOID FACTOR

Check the rheumatoid factor because it forms an integral part of mixed cryoglobulins.

• The IgM component of mixed cryoglobulins exhibits strong rheumatoid factor activity, which taken together with the low C4 is an important clue pointing towards mixed cryoglobulinaemia.
• By contrast, Wegener's granulomatosis and microscopic polyangiitis are characterized by normal or elevated complement levels as part of the acute phase response.

ANTINEUTROPHIL CYTOPLASMIC ANTIBODIES

Check antineutrophil cytoplasmic antibodies (ANCAs) in view of the possibility of Wegener's granulomatosis/microscopic polyangiitis.

Other tests

- Urine: dipstix for proteinuria and haematuria; microscopy of sediment for red cell casts as evidence of active glomerulonephritis.
- Renal function.
- Liver function: in view of the strong association between HCV and mixed cryoglobulinaemia.
- Check viral serology, especially hepatitis C. If negative, proceed to polymerase chain reaction (PCR) analysis of cyroprecipitate for HCV RNA.
- Renal biopsy: may be required to confirm the diagnosis and rule out other causes of renal dysfunction, e.g. drug-related interstitial nephritis. The glomerulonephritis in mixed cryoglobulinaemia has distinctive features, being characterized by marked deposition of immunoglobulin and complement (see Fig. 9). By contrast, a pauciimmune glomerulonephritis (little or no complement or immunoglobulin deposited in the glomeruli) would favour ANCA-positive systemic vasculitis.
- Chest radiograph: may show changes compatible with Wegener's granulomatosis; lung involvement is unusual in mixed cryoglobulinaemia.

Management

Mixed cryoglobulinaemia with hepatitis C infection

Interferon-α is the treatment of choice [3], although rapidly progressive disease may require immunosuppressive therapy (mycophenolate mofetil may be particularly indicated).

Idiopathic mixed cryoglobulinaemia with progressive renal or hepatic disease

Immunosuppressive therapy using steroids and cyclophosphamide or azathioprine. Plasmapheresis is a useful adjunct for the treatment of acute exacerbations, irrespective of the underlying aetiology.

See *Nephrology*, Sections 1.9, 1.12 and 2.7.
1 Lamprecht P, Gause A, Grass WL. Cryoglobulinaemic vasculitis (review). *Arthritis Rheumatism* 1999; 42: 2507–2516.
2 Misbah SA. Cryoglobulinaemia. In: *Oxford Textbook of Medicine*, 3rd edn (Weatherall D, Ledingham J, Warrell D, eds). Oxford: Oxford University Press, 1996.
3 Casato M, Agnello V, Pucillo LP *et al.* Predictors of long-term response to high-dose interferon therapy in type II cryoglobulinaemia associated with hepatitis C virus infection. *Blood* 1997; 90: 3865–3873.

1.11 Arthralgia and photosensitive rash

Case history

A 22-year-old woman presents with a 6-month history of joint pains and a photosensitive facial rash.

Clinical approach

Joint pains and a photosensitive rash in a young woman are very suggestive of systemic lupus erythematosus (SLE) (Fig. 10).

The following are other disorders that should be considered in cases of joint pain and skin rash:
- Viral infection*, e.g. parvovirus infection: may mimic SLE.
- Dermatomyositis: may present with arthralgia and a photosensitive rash in the 'V' of the neck and upper trunk.
- Lyme disease* and rheumatic fever*: characteristic skin rashes in association with arthralgia and systemic disease; should not cause difficulties in differential diagnosis.
- Psoriatic arthritis*.

*Photosensitivity is not a feature of these disorders; each has characteristic features that enable them to be

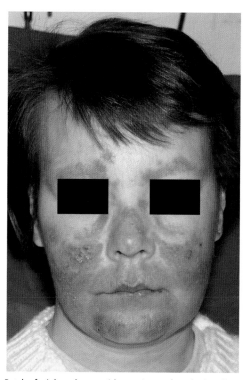

Fig. 10 Patchy facial erythema with scarring and marked eyebrow involvement in a patient with SLE. (Courtesy of Dr M Goodfield, Leeds General Infirmary.)

distinguished from SLE on clinical grounds. Proceed to serology in cases of diagnostic doubt.

History of the presenting problem

Is systemic lupus the explanation? The aim is to ask pertinent questions to clarify the presenting symptoms, in addition to relevant questions regarding involvement of other organ systems.

Affected joints

Ask about the following:
- Onset and course of pain.
- Distribution and symmetry: is it proximal or distal?
- Morning stiffness? This is a non-specific feature of any inflammatory joint disorder.

 Joint involvement occurs in 90% of patients with lupus and is characterized by a symmetrical, distal, non-erosive arthritis. Frank deforming arthritis is rare and occurs in a small minority of patients.

Nature of the rash

Ask about the distribution of the rash. Does it predominantly affect sun-exposed areas of the body? Does sunlight precipitate or aggravate the rash?

Skin manifestations of lupus may occur either on their own (discoid lupus erythematosus, subacute cutaneous lupus erythematosus) [1] or in association with systemic disease. In the latter situation, a photosensitive malar rash affecting the bridge of the nose and cheeks is characteristic.

Associated symptoms

Ask about the following, which are pointers towards the diagnosis and activity of lupus:
- Hair loss
- Livedo reticularis
- Raynaud's phenomenon
- Mouth ulcers
- Chest or abdominal pain (serositis?), dyspnoea
- Headaches
- Seizures
- Drug history to exclude possibility of drug-induced lupus.

Examination

- General: note the type and distribution of rash. Also look for pallor, lymphadenopathy, mouth ulcers and alopecia, all of which might be present in lupus.

- Joints: examine the joints in a logical sequence of 'look', 'feel' and 'move'. Is there synovitis? Joints with significant synovitis are painful and have a limited range of movement.
- Chest and heart: Listen for pleural or pericardial rubs. Check blood pressure.
- Nervous system: detailed neurological examination is not required in most cases, but check for gross long tract deficits and peripheral neuropathy, and examine the fundi for exudates.

Approach to investigations and management

Investigations

Immunological

ANTIBODIES TO NUCLEAR ANTIGENS (ANA, DNA, ENA)

As SLE is the main diagnosis under consideration, the patient's ANA status is crucial.

 Using human epithelial cells (HEp-2) as a substrate, ANA positivity (titre ≥1 : 80) occurs in >99% of patients with untreated SLE. Conversely, a negative ANA effectively excludes systemic lupus [2].

As a positive ANA can occur in a variety of other disorders, it is important to characterize its specificity, i.e. is it directed against double-stranded DNA and/or other extractable nuclear antigens (ENA—individual specificities known as Ro, La, Sm, RNP)?

 Antibodies to DNA and ENA are specific for lupus or lupus overlap disorders, and occur in 30–90% of patients.

SERUM COMPLEMENT LEVELS

Check C3 and C4 levels. Patients with lupus may be hypocomplementaemic as a result of active disease and/or possession of one or more C4 null alleles.

ANTIPHOSPHOLIPID ANTIBODIES

Check for anticardiolipin antibodies and lupus anticoagulant. These antibodies occur in 30% of lupus patients and act as markers for thrombosis (Fig. 11).

Other tests

Check the following:
- Urine: dipstix for proteinuria and haematuria;

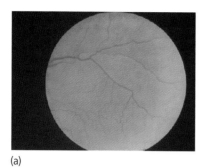

(a)

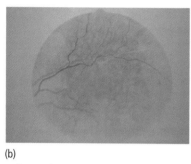

(b)

Fig. 11 (a) Branch retinal artery occlusion in a patient with SLE and the antiphospholipid syndrome; the defect is more pronounced in the subtraction angiogram (b).

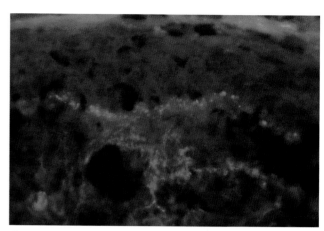

Fig. 12 Granular IgG deposits at the dermoepidermal junction (lupus band). (Courtesy of Dr W Merchant, Leeds General Infirmary.)

microscopy of sediment for red cell casts as evidence of active glomerulonephritis.

- Renal function.
- Liver function.
- Full blood count (FBC): looking for cytopenia.
- C-reactive protein (CRP): marker of inflammation/infection. This is often normal in active uncomplicated lupus [3] despite an elevated erythrocyte sedimentation rate (ESR) or plasma viscosity.

If SLE is confirmed:

- Document baseline renal function more precisely with 24-h urinary collection for protein and creatinine clearance. If renal function is significantly impaired (creatinine >140 μmol/L or proteinuria >1 g/24 h), it is likely that a renal biopsy will be required to determine prognosis and guide treatment decisions.
- Skin biopsies are seldom performed in the assessment of SLE, although the demonstration of a 'lupus band' is useful in the diagnosis of cutaneous LE (Fig. 12).

Management

Systemic lupus erythematosus

MILD DISEASE

Mild disease confined to the skin and joints responds well to chloroquine, non-steroidal anti-inflammatory drugs (NSAIDs) and low-dose steroids either singly or in combination.

SEVERE DISEASE

Severe lupus with major organ involvement (kidneys and brain) requires more powerful immunosuppressive therapy using steroids and cyclophosphamide [4].

PHOSPHOLIPID SYNDROME

Patients with the phospholipid syndrome require prophylactic antithrombotic therapy.

ALL CASES

Long-term follow-up with regular monitoring of disease activity is essential. Do not forget general advice regarding sun exposure, potential problems of long-term steroids and oestrogen-based contraception.

SLE excluded

Management is the symptomatic treatment of arthralgia and rash.

See Section 1.12, pp. 25–26.
See *Dermatology*, Sections 1.4 and 1.6.
See *Haematology*, Sections 1.8, 1.13 and 2.4.
See *Nephrology*, Sections 1.9 and 2.7.5.

1 McCauliffe D. Distinguishing subacute cutaneous from other types of lupus erythematosus. *Lancet* 1998; 351: 1527–1528.
2 Wallace DJ, Linker-Israeli M. It's not the same old lupus or Sjögren's any more: one hundred new insights, approaches, and options since 1990. *Curr Opin Rheumatol* 1999; 11: 321–329.
3 Kushner I. C-reactive protein in rheumatology. *Arthritis Rheum* 1991; 34: 1065–1068.
4 JA Mills. Systemic lupus erythematosus. *N Engl J Med* 1994; 330: 1871–1879.

1.12 Systemic lupus erythematosus and confusion

Case history

A 35-year-old woman with a 2-year history of known SLE presents in an acute confusional state.

Clinical approach

Neurological symptoms in a patient with SLE merit urgent investigation. Your aim is to distinguish between the following [1]:
- Neuropsychiatric SLE
- Central nervous system (or other) infection in an immunocompromised individual
- A side effect of drug (steroid) treatment
- Unrelated neurological/psychiatric illness.

It can be very difficult indeed to do this, but very important because the treatment of these entities is radically different.

History of the presenting problem

Neuropsychiatric SLE

Neurological involvement in lupus usually occurs on a background of active systemic disease but may occasionally occur anew. You should ask relevant questions to assess whether her lupus is active (see Section 1.11, p. 23). If the patient is incapable of coherent conversation, ask a relative or partner.

Other neurological/psychiatric symptoms

Neuropsychiatric SLE may present with diffuse or focal symptoms. Ask about the following:
- Headache
- Seizures
- Problems with vision
- Limb weakness
- Psychotic symptoms.

Existing drugs

It is important to find out what drugs the patient is taking now, and what she has been given over the last 2 years since her lupus was diagnosed. This is important because it may provide diagnostic clues:
- Someone who has been given pulsed methylprednisolone, cyclophosphamide and other 'aggressive' treatments is clearly prone to immunosuppression-related infection.

- Someone who has received only a modest dose of steroids, perhaps with azathioprine, is at much less risk.

 Opportunistic infection may masquerade as neuropsychiatric SLE in patients on prolonged immunosuppressive therapy, and a recent increase in her steroid dosage may suggest steroid-induced psychosis.

Relevant past history

Has anything like this happened before? Is there any history of psychiatric disorder?

Examination

Is the patient well, unwell, very ill or near death? If near death, call for help from the intensive care unit (ICU) immediately. Check vital signs, Glasgow Coma Score (GCS) and Abbreviated Mental Test (AMT) score. Begin resuscitation immediately if this is necessary (see *Emergency medicine*, Section 1.2).

Look carefully for evidence of lupus activity, as described in Section 1.11, pp. 22–24. Additional emphasis is required on the neurological examination, taking particular care to look for the following:
- Meningism
- Fundi for papilloedema, exudates
- Cranial and peripheral nerves for mononeuritis multiplex
- Limbs for evidence of transverse myelitis.

Approach to investigations and management

This will be dictated by the nature of the presentation. The differential diagnosis of an acute confusional state is very wide. If the patient looks as though she has a sepsis syndrome, e.g. cool or warm peripheries, hypotension, high fever, then she should be treated accordingly, acknowledging that the differential diagnosis will be wider than usual in someone who is immunosuppressed. Neuropsychiatric SLE does not cause circulatory compromise.

This woman's vital signs were not grossly abnormal: temperature, 37.4°C, pulse 80/min, respiration 14/min; her peripheral circulation was normal and pulse oximetry showed an oxygen saturation of 98% on air. Her GCS was 13/15 and her AMT score 6/10. Neurological examination was difficult, but there were no clear focal signs and no meningism.

Investigation

Immunological

 Note that there is no single reliable laboratory or radiological marker of neuropsychiatric SLE [2]. A combination of serum, CSF and imaging studies yields the highest diagnostic yield. Clinical acumen is therefore paramount in diagnosing neuropsychiatric SLE.

SEROLOGY

Urgent serology is required to assess lupus activity. Check ANA, antibodies to double-stranded DNA, complement C3 and C4 levels and CRP. Antineuronal and antiribosomal P antibodies have been promoted as markers of neuropsychiatric SLE but are rarely used in practice because of a combination of methodological difficulties and poor sensitivity. Although many cases of neuropsychiatric SLE are associated with worsening serology, exceptional cases may occur with stable serology. A raised CRP is unusual in lupus itself (see Section 1.11, pp. 22–24) and should raise suspicions of infection.

ANTIPHOSPHOLIPID ANTIBODIES

Antiphospholipid antibodies (anticardiolipin and lupus anticoagulant) are useful in delineating patients with the phospholipid syndrome, who may present with confusion secondary to thrombotic disease.

Other tests

The following will be required:
• Dipstix urine for protein and blood: if positive, microscope urine for red cell casts. Has she got active lupus nephritis? If she has, this would make neuropsychiatric SLE more likely.
• Check FBC, electrolytes, renal and liver function tests, blood cultures, urine cultures.
• Image the brain: a gadolinium-enhanced MR scan would be the preferred test, but if not available rapidly then proceed to contrast-enhanced CT scan.
• Lumbar puncture: perform as soon as imaging has excluded raised intracranial pressure/mass effect.

 Urgent imaging to clarify underlying cerebral pathology and exclude space-occupying lesions. A gadolinium-enhanced MRI scan is the imaging modality of choice but note that a negative scan does not rule out CNS lupus [2].
  Examination of CSF is essential to exclude opportunistic infection. A non-specific cellular pleiocytosis, rise in protein and CSF oligoclonal bands occur in 30% of cases.

Management

Neuropsychiatric SLE requires aggressive immunosuppressive therapy using parenteral steroids and cyclophosphamide. If infection cannot be excluded, use concomitant antimicrobial therapy. Opportunistic CNS infection should be treated appropriately.

 See *Medicine for the elderly*, Section 1.2.
See *Emergency medicine*, Sections 1.26 and 1.28.
See *Infectious diseases*, Sections 1.16, 1.17 and sections on specific pathogens.
1 Hanly JG. Evaluation of patients with CNS involvement in SLE. *Baillière's Clin Rheumatol* 1998; 12: 415–431.
2 ACR nomenclature and case definitions for neuropsychiatric lupus syndromes. *Arthritis Rheum* 1999; 42: 599–608.

1.13 Cold fingers and difficulty in swallowing

Case history

You are asked to see a 50-year-old woman with a 9-month history of cold fingers and recent difficulty in swallowing.

Clinical approach

It is important to clarify both these symptoms because cold fingers might mean different things to different people, and the meaning of difficulty in swallowing may range from occasional benign choking to true dysphagia. The following are key questions to consider:
• Are her cold fingers as a result of Raynaud's phenomenon? If so, is this a primary problem or secondary to underlying connective tissue disease (Table 10)?
• If the diagnosis is scleroderma, is it the result of a diffuse or limited cutaneous type of systemic sclerosis? Is there evidence of visceral involvement?

 Causes of secondary Raynaud's phenomenon
• Connective tissue diseases: scleroderma, SLE, rheumatoid arthritis, inflammatory myositis.
• Occlusive arterial disease: thoracic outlet syndrome, atherosclerosis/embolism, thromboangiitis obliterans.
• Occupational: vibrating tools.
• Drugs: ergotamine, β blockers and polyvinyl chloride.
• Intravascular coagulation or aggregation: cryoglobulinaemia, cold agglutinin disease and polycythaemia rubra vera.

Table 10 Comparison of primary and secondary Raynaud's phenomenon.

Characteristics	Primary Raynaud's phenomenon	Secondary Raynaud's phenomenon
Age (average) (years)	30	>50
Sex	Female	Female
Tissue damage	Absent	Digital ulcers, gangrene
Symmetry	Symmetrical attacks	Asymmetrical attacks
Capillaroscopy	Negative	Positive
Antinuclear antibody	Negative	Positive
Associated disease	No associated disease	Scleroderma, SLE, lupus overlap

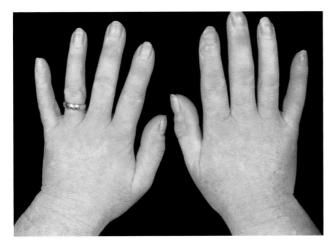

Fig. 13 Finger pallor during an attack of Raynaud's phenomenon.

History of presenting problem

Are the cold fingers caused by Raynaud's phenomenon? Consider the following, which also help to distinguish primary from secondary causes:
• Is there colour change? Pallor, cyanosis and rubor are the typical triphasic colour changes of Raynaud's phenomenon, although many patients will describe only biphasic changes.
• Where? Usually in the fingers (Fig. 13), but other areas affected are toes and ears.
• How bad and for how long?
• Is it associated with trophic changes/ulcers in the fingers?
• What are the precipitating factors? Raynaud's phenomenon is usually provoked by exposure to cold and emotional stress and terminated by rewarming, or it may abate spontaneously.

Obstruction of major arteries

Consider obstruction of major upper arm arteries (atherosclerosis, thrombosis and embolism), which may mimic Raynaud's phenomenon:
• Colour changes may be similar to those in Raynaud's phenomenon
• Symptoms are more likely to be unilateral
• Arm claudication is characteristic
• Low blood pressure and reduced peripheral pulses in the affected arm
• Arteriography demonstrates the arterial lesion.

Does the patient have one of the causes of secondary Raynaud's phenomenon? Assess the following:
• Dysphagia (see *Gastroenterology and hepatology*, Sections 1.2 and 2.2)
• Symptoms of other connective tissue disorders: arthralgia/arthritis, photosensitivity, rashes, alopecia and proximal muscle weakness
• Review of other systems: respiratory, cardiac and gastrointestinal
• Drug history
• Occupation
• Family history of connective tissue disease
• Smoking.

Examination

Look particularly at the following:
• Skin: is there a characteristic butterfly rash or telangiectasias on the cheeks. Check for tight skin, Gottron's patches (Fig. 14) and calcinosis.
• Supraclavicular fossa for tenderness or mass (possible cervical rib).
• Joints: evidence of arthritis.
• Cardiovascular: check pulses and blood pressure in both arms, neck bruits and cardiac murmurs.

Approach to investigations and management

Raynaud's phenomenon

Check the following
• FBC: patients with secondary Raynaud's phenomenon may be anaemic as a result of chronic disease itself, gastrointestinal blood loss and/or malabsorption.
• Urine dipstix for protein and blood (with urine microscopy if positive) and renal function: abnormalities would not be expected in primary Raynaud's phenomenon and would suggest renal problems related to a secondary disorder.
• Inflammatory markers: the ESR and CRP are usually normal in primary Raynaud's phenomenon, but may be elevated in secondary Raynaud's phenomenon if there is tissue damage.
• Antinuclear antibodies: typically negative in primary Raynaud's phenomenon.

• Nail-fold capillary microscopy: useful in differentiating primary from secondary Raynaud's phenomenon. Abnormal nail-fold capillary morphology indicates secondary disease and predicts the presence or future development of connective tissue disease.

Five per cent of the general population have Raynaud's phenomenon, yet only a minority eventually develop an associated connective tissue disease. The following are the frequencies of Raynaud's phenomenon in those with autoimmune rheumatic disease:
• Scleroderma: 95%
• SLE: 20%
• Sjögren's syndrome: 20%
• Myositis: 20%
• Rheumatoid arthritis: 5%.
A positive ANA in a patient with Raynaud's phenomenon is predictive of underlying connective tissue disease; positive centromere or anti-Scl 70 antibodies are predictive of the CREST (**c**alcinosis, **R**aynaud's, **o**esophageal dysfunction, **s**clerodactyly, **t**elangiectasia) syndrome or scleroderma.

Management

See Section 2.4.3, p. 88.

See *Gastroenterology and hepatology*, Sections 1.2, 1.10 and 2.2.
Grassi W, de-Angelis R, Lapadula G *et al.* Clinical diagnoses found in patients with Raynaud's phenomenon. *Rheumatol Int* 1998; 18: 17–20.
Ho M, Belch JJ. Raynaud's phenomenon: state of the art 1998 (review). *Scand J Rheumatol* 1998; 27: 319–322.
Isenberg DA, Black C. Raynaud's phenomenon, scleroderma and overlap syndromes. *BMJ* 1995; 310: 795–798.

1.14 Dry eyes and fatigue

Case history

A middle-aged woman presents with a history of fatigue, dry mouth, dry eyes and bilateral parotid swelling. Initial investigations reveal a raised ESR (60 mm/h), a positive ANA at a titre of 1 : 640 and positive rheumatoid factor.

Clinical approach

Her symptoms constitute the sicca complex (keratoconjunctivitis and xerostomia). On a background of parotid enlargement, raised ESR, positive ANA and rheumatoid factor, this is likely to result from Sjögren's syndrome. The syndrome may occur by itself (primary Sjögren's syndrome) or on a background of connective tissue disease [1].

Table 11 Differential diagnosis of bilateral parotid enlargement.

Disorder	Comments
Viral infection (mumps, EBV, Coxackie A, CMV, HIV)	Usually acute in onset on a background of systemic ill-health
Sarcoidosis	Occurs on a background of systemic disease
Sjögren's syndrome	Positive ANA, rheumatoid factor, antibodies to Ro and La
Miscellaneous group: diabetes, hyperlipidaemia, alcohol abuse, acromegaly, chronic renal failure	Other clues to primary diagnosis usually present

CMV, cytomegalovirus; EBV, Epstein–Barr virus; HIV, human immunodeficiency virus.

Alternative causes of parotid enlargement (Table 11) here should be considered in the differential diagnosis, but these rarely cause diagnostic confusion.

History of the presenting problem

Assess the severity of her sicca symptoms by asking the following questions:
• Do you feel a gritty sensation in your eyes?
• Do you have sore eyes or difficulty in wearing contact lenses?
• Do you have difficulty in trying to eat dry foods (cracker sign)?
• Do you need to take liquids to aid swallowing?
• Do you wake up at night with a dry mouth and have to take sips of water?
   Enquire about other important symptoms:
• Joint pain and swelling: active synovitis may be a feature of primary Sjögren's syndrome or indicate associated diseases such as rheumatoid arthritis or lupus.
• Raynaud's phenomenon is seen in 20% of cases of primary Sjögren's syndrome (also common in secondary Sjögren's syndrome).
• Purpuric rash indicating cutaneous vasculitis may occur in up to 30% of patients.

Sjögren's syndrome may frequently be asymptomatic in middle-aged women, manifesting with a persistently elevated ESR or plasma viscosity (with normal CRP) accompanied by polyclonal hypergammaglobulinaemia and antibodies to Ro and La antigens.

Examination

Examine the following:
• Eyes: conjunctival congestion and dried secretions along the inner canthus
• Mouth: dry tongue, angular cheilitis, dental caries

- Enlarged parotid glands (fullness behind the ear lobes)
- Skin: purpura (usually in the lower limb)
- Musculoskeletal system: arthritis and signs of other connective tissue diseases
- Chest: fine basal crepitations (pulmonary fibrosis)
- Abdomen: hepatosplenomegaly and features of chronic liver disease; primary biliary cirrhosis is a recognized association
- Neurological assessment: peripheral neuropathy and cranial nerve lesions (trigeminal neuralgia).

Approach to investigations and management

Investigations to confirm Sjögren's syndrome

- Schirmer's tear test to obtain objective evidence of reduced tear secretion using strips of filter paper inserted into the lower eyelid. Wetting of less than 5 mm in 5 min is considered pathological. (See Section 2.4.2, p. 85.)
- Keratoconjunctivitis sicca, a consequence of reduced tear production, is diagnosed using rose bengal staining of the cornea.
- Check ANA and antibodies to Ro and La antigens: these are present in 40–90% of patients with Sjögren's syndrome. (See Section 3.2, pp. 98–101.)
- Minor salivary gland biopsy for histological evidence of focal lymphocytic infiltrates. In practice, biopsies are rarely required in view of the ease with which antibodies to Ro and La can be detected [2].
- Severity of xerostomia can be assessed using salivary gland scintigraphy and sialometry, but both of these investigations are rarely performed in routine practice.

Potential sources of diagnostic confusion when performing Schirmer's test:
- Concomitant anticholinergic therapy
- Old age.

Other investigations

Check the following:
- Thyroid function: in view of the strong association between Sjögren's syndrome and hypothyroidism.
- Inflammatory markers: the ESR is usually persistently elevated as a direct consequence of polyclonal hyper-gammaglobulinaemia; by contrast, the CRP is often normal
- Rheumatoid factor: positive in 90%
- Complement: C3 and C4 levels are usually normal in Sjögren's syndrome; consider mixed cryoglobulinaemia if C4 is low [3].

Management

Therapy for Sjögren's syndrome is limited to symptomatic relief and limitation of the damaging local effects of the sicca complex using the following:
- Artificial tears, sugar-free candies and chewing gum
- Meticulous dental hygiene
- Avoidance of diuretics and anticholinergic agents.

Immunosuppressive therapy is of little value in uncomplicated Sjögren's syndrome.

1 Venables PJ. Sjögren's syndrome. In: Weatherall D, Ledingham J, Warrell D, eds. *Oxford Textbook of Medicine*, 3rd edn. Oxford: Oxford University Press, 1996: 3036–3038.
2 Fox RI, Tornwall J, Michelson P. Current issues in the diagnosis and treatment of Sjögren's syndrome. *Curr Opin Rheumatol* 1999; 11: 364–371.
3 Ramos-Casals M, Cervera R, Yague J *et al.* Cryoglobulinaemia in primary Sjögren's syndrome: prevalence and clinical characteristics in a series of 115 patients. *Semin Arthritis Rheum* 1998; 28: 200–205.

1.15 Breathlessness and weakness

Case history

A 35-year-old woman presents with a 6-week history of breathlessness, aching thighs and shoulders, and insidiously progressive weakness. She now finds it difficult to climb stairs and rise from a low chair.

Clinical approach

The history raises an immediate suspicion of a proximal myopathy. This should trigger a hierarchy of diagnostic questions. Is the weakness real—or could the primary problem be pain rather than weakness? Weakness is usually more prominent than pain in primary muscle disease. Is this true proximal weakness—or could there be another cause of symmetrical leg weakness, e.g. spinal cord pathology?

If a myopathic pattern of weakness is present, consider the diagnoses listed in Table 12. If dermatomyositis or polymyositis is likely [1]:
- Consider a search for associated malignancy
- Remember to be alert for non-muscular manifestations of connective tissue disease.

Disorder type	Disorder	Comments
Inflammatory (idiopathic)	Polymyositis/dermatomyositis	Associated with rash and features of autoimmune rheumatic disorder, also with malignancy
		See text for further discussion
	Polymyalgia rheumatica	>55 years only
		Weakness secondary to pain
		General malaise
		Anaemia of chronic disorders
		Raised inflammatory markers
		No other organ involvement
		Negative serological tests
Endocrine/metabolic	Cushing's syndrome	Look for associated features of steroid excess
		Exogenous steroids are a very common cause of proximal myopathy
	Thyrotoxicosis	Look for associated features
		Check thyroid function tests
	Osteomalacia	Rare in this age group, when likely to be the result of malabsorption
	Diabetes mellitus	Diabetic amyotrophy affects the quadriceps, causing pain and weakness
		Usually asymmetrical
		Does not affect shoulder girdle
Other	Myasthenia gravis	Critical clinical feature is fatiguability
	Carcinomatous neuromyopathy	Usually found in patients with known malignancy, but can be a presenting feature
	Trichinella spiralis	Acquired from eating improperly cooked pork
		Weakness caused by muscular pain, a feature of the larval migration stage

Table 12 Causes of proximal muscle weakness developing over a few weeks.

In suspected myositis think about:
• Alternative causes of weakness
• Malignancy
• Changes in other systems, especially the lungs.

History of the presenting problem

Gain a picture of the pattern of symptoms and their rate of progression:

• When did the weakness start? A very long history might suggest an inherited muscle dystrophy presenting in an adult. Although the history is said to be of 6 weeks' duration, could it be longer than this? A year ago, could she walk as far and as fast as other people? Has she ever been able to do this?

• What are the functional consequences of the weakness? Can the woman get up stairs at all and, if so, how does she do it? Can she brush her hair? Is there anything to suggest defective control of swallowing or the upper airway? Has she choked when drinking?

• Is pain a prominent feature? If it is, this might indicate osteomalacia or fibromyalgia.

• Does the history suggest rapid onset of fatigue with repeated movement, possibly as a result of myasthenia (see *Neurology*, Section 2.2.5)?

• Are there any other neurological symptoms, particularly sensory changes that would suggest a non-myopathic cause?

• Ask specifically about the breathlessness. Is exercise limited by weakness of the legs or by the breathing? Breathing difficulty could be caused by myopathy of the respiratory muscles or be associated with lung disease (alveolitis).

If information does not emerge spontaneously, ask about the following, which may give important clues about a systemic disorder. Think about the conditions listed in Table 12 as you do so:

• General: weight loss or weight gain, preference for hot or cold weather—these could be clues to malignancy, Cushing's syndrome or thyrotoxicosis.

• Skin: has there been a rash, especially a photosensitive rash, which might be found in both SLE and dermatomyositis?

• Joints: has there been any pain or swelling?

• Hands: does the woman have Raynaud's phenomenon?

- Eyes and mouth: any problems with gritty eyes or dry mouth? These might suggest presentation of Sjögren's syndrome (see Section 1.14, pp. 28–29).
- Respiratory: has there been pleuritic pain or haemoptysis?
- Gastrointestinal: have there been any new symptoms?
- Neurological: this woman is too young but, in an older patient, have there been headaches that might indicate temporal arteritis/polymyalgia rheumatica?
- Pregnancy history: multiple fetal losses might indicate the presence of antiphospholipid antibody.
- Previous vascular or thromboembolic disease: might indicate the presence of antiphospholipid antibody.

Examination

General

Assess the general state of the patient. If he or she appears very unwell, consider severe respiratory failure, aspiration pneumonia or underlying malignancy. Is there anything to suggest thyroid disease or Cushing's syndrome? A thorough examination of all systems is required, but concentrate on the following.

Skin

Is the skin abnormal? The typical rash of dermatomyositis is photosensitive in distribution, often scaly (Gottron's papules—Fig. 14), and often associated with marked subcutaneous oedema (especially around the eyes). Nail-fold capillaries are often visibly enlarged. Other rashes that may be seen are those of lupus.

 Look at the hands—puffy fingers and active vasospasm suggest scleroderma or mixed connective tissue disease.

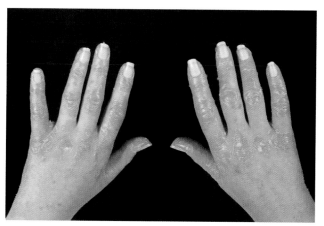

Fig. 14 Scaly patches (known as Gottron's papules) on the dorsal surface of the hands in dermatomyositis.

Neurological

Neurological assessment should focus on determining whether or not true proximal weakness is present, and looking carefully for features that would suggest diagnoses other than myopathy as the cause of leg weakness:
- Fasciculation and long tract signs (motor neuron disease?)
- Sensory changes in the hands, long tract signs in the legs (myelopathy?)
- Distal weakness and areflexia (Guillain–Barré?)
- Diplopia, bulbar weakness and fatiguability (myasthenia?).

Malignancy

Look carefully for evidence of malignancy:
- Weight loss/cachexia
- Clubbing
- Lymphadenopathy
- Breast, abdominal and pelvic masses (consider especially ovarian malignancy)
- Abnormal chest signs that may suggest pulmonary fibrosis, pneumonia or malignancy.

Approach to investigations and management

Investigations

The diagnosis may be clear from the history and examination, in which case investigations should be appropriately tailored; otherwise, the following issues need to be addressed.

Muscle disease

- Creatine kinase (CK) estimation is the most useful marker of muscle damage. However, myopathies may occur with a normal CK, and the CK may be raised in the absence of muscle disease (e.g. after heavy exercise).
- Other enzymes (such as aspartate transaminase [AST] and alanine transaminase [ALT]) may be raised, leading to the potential for confusion with liver disease if myopathy is not initially suspected.
- Electromyography provides useful evidence to confirm myopathy and to exclude denervation as a cause of weakness.
- Muscle biopsy remains the only tool for definitive differential diagnosis of myopathy.
- Magnetic resonance imaging is useful in patchy myositis to identify a site for biopsy.

Identifying the underlying cause

The extent of investigation for malignancy is determined by clinical suspicion and the patient's age. A minimal screen would be a chest radiograph and abdominal and pelvic ultrasonography.

Endocrinological investigation (for steroid excess and vitamin D studies) should be considered, depending on the clinical picture.

Are immunological markers of inflammatory myositis present? Consider appropriate tests in suspected lupus and other connective tissue diseases (see Sections 1.11, pp. 22–24 and 3.2, pp. 98–101). Antibodies to Jo-1 (histidyl-tRNA synthetase) occur in 30–50% of patients with dermatomyositis and polymyositis and act as a marker for interstitial lung disease.

Antibodies to Jo-1

Antibodies to Jo-1 identify a distinct group of patients with inflammatory myositis, designated the anti-synthetase syndrome (myositis, fever, interstitial lung disease, Raynaud's phenomenon, symmetrical non-erosive arthritis) [2].

Management

Beware of respiratory failure in patients severely affected by polymyositis/dermatomyositis. Swallowing and the airway may be compromised with the risk of aspiration. Any patient with severe muscular weakness will require physiotherapy to minimize wasting and prevent contractures. Management otherwise depends on the cause. Treatment of inflammatory muscle disease is with corticosteroids and immunosuppressants.

See *Endocrinology*, Section 1.16.
See *Emergency medicine*, Section 1.23.
See *Neurology*, Sections 1.13, 2.1.3, 2.2, 2.2.5, 2.11.1 and 3.3.
1 Callen JP. Dermatomyositis. *Lancet* 2000; 355: 53–57.
2 Plotz PH. Myositis: immunological contributions to understanding cause, pathogenesis and therapy (NIH Conference). *Ann Intern Med* 1995; 122: 715–724.

1.16 Prolonged fever and joint pains

Case history

A 20-year-old woman presents with a 6-week history of high fever, sore throat and joint pains. Extensive investigation in hospital is largely unrewarding except for a normochromic/normocytic anaemia, with a markedly raised ESR at 100 mm/L, CRP at 200 mg/L (normal <10 mg/L) and a plasma ferritin at 5000 μg/L (normal <300 μL). Negative or normal investigations comprise the following:

Table 13 Differential diagnosis of fever and arthritis.

Infection	Direct invasion: bacterial (mycobacterial), fungal, Whipple's disease
	Indirect: bacterial (acute rheumatic fever), reactive arthritis
Crystal arthropathy	Urate
	Calcium pyrophosphate
Inflammatory disorders	Lupus and lupus overlap disorders
	Necrotizing vasculitis
	Adult-onset Still's disease
	Rheumatoid arthritis
	Sarcoidosis
	Arthritis associated with inflammatory bowel disease
Haematological malignancies	

Modified from Van De Putte LBA, Wouters JM. Adult-onset Still's disease. *Bailliére's Clin Rheumatol* 1991; 2: 263–275.

- Anti-streptolysin titre
- Blood and urine cultures
- Autoantibodies: ANA, ANCA, rheumatoid factor
- Serum angiotensin-converting enzyme
- Chest radiograph
- CT scan of thorax, abdomen and pelvis
- Bone marrow biopsy: culture for acid- and alcohol-fast bacilli
- Transthoracic echocardiography.

Clinical approach

Prolonged fever with joint pains has a wide differential diagnosis, covering a range of inflammatory, infective and neoplastic conditions (Table 13). A thorough history is therefore crucial. The negative ANA effectively excludes systemic lupus and related disorders (see Section 1.11, pp. 22–24), but the negative rheumatoid factor is of little help in confirming or excluding rheumatoid arthritis. The patient's markedly raised CRP and ESR would fit with either an inflammatory or an infective disorder.

The crucial clue in this case is the long list of negative investigations, which in this clinical setting points to adult Still's disease as a likely cause [1].

History of the presenting problem

Systemic Still's disease

Adult Still's disease is an acute systemic inflammatory disorder that poses a diagnostic challenge because of the lack of pathognomonic clinical or laboratory features [2]. Ask about the following:

- Onset and frequency of fever

• Onset and distribution of joint pain: polyarthralgia affecting the knees, wrists and fingers is common, with some patients developing frank arthritis with sterile effusions.
• Sore throat is a common feature of Still's disease, but uncommon in other systemic inflammatory disorders.
• Rashes: a fleeting rash is a useful diagnostic clue, although it may be misinterpreted as a drug allergy because penicillin is often given for the sore throat.
• Pain compatible with pleurisy or pericarditis: both are features of adult Still's disease.

 Still's disease is characterized by high spiking fever ('sawtooth' pattern) accompanied by pronounced myalgia, arthralgia and sweats.

Examination

Thorough examinations will no doubt have been performed, but don't rely on this, and look in particular for the following:
• Rash: what type and what distribution?
• Lymphadenopathy, hepatomegaly and splenomegaly: all are features of adult Still's disease.
• Joints: is there evidence of synovitis?
• Muscle tenderness and weakness: a true myositis with raised muscle enzymes is exceptional and should suggest an alternative diagnosis in a patient with suspected Still's disease.

Approach to investigations and management

Investigations

In the absence of a specific marker, the diagnosis of adult Still's disease is entirely based on clinical grounds.

Detailed laboratory investigations and appropriate imaging are essential to exclude infections, autoimmune rheumatic disease (see Section 1.11, pp. 22–24) and haematological malignancy. Neutrophil counts and inflammatory markers are raised: marked hyperferritinaemia between 1500 and 10 000 µg/L (normal <300 µg/L) is a feature in >90% of patients and correlates with disease activity. Although ferritin is a non-specific acute phase protein, the magnitude of its rise in this clinical setting is a useful pointer to adult Still's disease.

 The 'classic triad' occurs in <50% of patients with adult Still's disease:
• Arthritis
• Persistent spiking fever
• A fleeting maculopapular rash.
Virtually all patients with adult Still's disease have markedly elevated ESR, CRP and neutrophil counts. Serum ferritin levels are usually very high.

Management

Aspirin and other non-steroidal anti-inflammatory agents have traditionally been considered as first-line therapy but are successful in only 20% of cases. Over 50% of patients require long-term steroid treatment.

 See *Infectious diseases*, Section 1.10.
1 Evans RH. Pyrexia of unknown origin (grand round). *BMJ* 1997; 314: 583–586.
2 Mok CC, Lau CS, Wong RWS. Clinical characteristics, treatment and outcome of adult onset Still's disease in Southern Chinese. *J Rheumatol* 1998; 25: 2345–2351.

1.17 Back pain

Case histories

Case A

A 35-year-old man presents with severe low back pain, which has forced him to give up working as a plasterer. The pain began in his late teens, was initially episodic, and was improved by rest and provoked by standing or stooping. On occasions the pain was associated with right-sided sciatica, but not with any motor or sensory disturbance. Over the years the episodes of pain became longer until he was never free from pain. His sleep is now disturbed and he is increasingly depressed and frustrated.

Case B

A 21-year-old man presents with severe low back pain. This began insidiously in his mid-teens and has slowly worsened since then. His back feels stiff and restricted each morning, but becomes looser and more comfortable as the day goes on. His chest wall aches and, in recent months, his neck has also displayed a similar pattern of pain. Two years ago he developed an acutely painful red right eye and an ophthalmologist made a diagnosis of acute anterior uveitis.

Case C

A 35-year-old woman presents with a 24-h history of low back pain radiating to both legs and a 6-h history of progressive numbness involving the back of the legs and then the perineum.

Table 14 The main serious and progressive back pain syndromes.

Disorder	Examples
Neoplastic	Common causes: lung, breast, prostate, myeloma
Infective	Discitis or epidural abscess—TB or bacterial
Inflammatory	Ankylosing spondylitis
Neurological	Cauda equina compression usually caused by tumour or disc prolapse

Case D

A 65-year-old man presents with severe mid-thoracic pain of 6 weeks' duration. The pain is progressive and is now disturbing his sleep. He has lost around a stone (6.3 kg) in weight since the pain developed.

Clinical approach

The challenge in assessment of back pain is to sort the wood from the trees using clinical acumen. A very small proportion of patients have serious, progressive pathology and need rapid access to appropriate investigations and management (Table 14). A more significant minority have back pain with referred leg pain caused by a variable degree of nerve root entrapment, usually as a result of disc prolapse. This often settles spontaneously but may require investigation and intervention. The majority of patients, however, have mechanical back pain and require little or no investigation—they are best served by a rehabilitative approach with minimal medical intervention [1].

This section refers mainly to the lower back, but in general the same approach can be applied to cervical pain. Thoracic pain is more unusual, reflecting the relative immobility of this part of the spine, and new or progressive pain in this area should always raise concerns about serious pathology.

History of the presenting problem

Type of pain

The pattern of the pain is critical. Mechanical back pain usually begins between the ages of 20 and 40, is initially episodic and of rapid onset, and each episode is usually precipitated by movement, although not necessarily by heavy lifting. This pattern may shift over time to continuous pain, often with superimposed exacerbations. The pain is typically worsened by activity and often (but not always) relieved by rest, but this may not be the case, especially in chronic back pain.

Beware of sudden onset of pain in a patient who might be osteoporotic because this may point to a crush fracture (see Section 1.23, pp. 47–49). Subacute progressive pain, particularly if there is no previous history, raises concerns

about a serious inflammatory or neoplastic cause. So-called red flag features can be used to help identify these patients.

Red flag features in back pain

- Age >55 or <18 years
- Progressive pain
- Night pain
- Systemic symptoms such as weight loss
- Progressive neurological defect
- Past history of malignancy or immunosuppression
- Recent trauma.

Neurological symptoms

The presence of neurological symptoms will usually be volunteered but should be actively sought.

Unilateral nerve root compression

Unilateral nerve root compression is indicated by the following:
- Referred pain with radicular distribution
- Lower limb dermatomal sensory disturbance
- Lower limb motor disturbance.

Cauda equina compression

Evidence of cauda equina compression includes the following:
- Bilateral leg pain
- Altered perineal sensation
- Bladder or bowel dysfunction.

Other medical clues

Consider the diagnoses listed in Table 14: are there any clues to support one of these diagnoses?

Psychological or psychiatric features

Assessment of the patient's degree of psychological distress is important. Depression is commonly seen in chronic pain and is an important factor in its perpetuation. Psychosocial yellow flags can be used to help identify the patient with poor prognosis from mechanical back pain.

Psychosocial yellow flags
- Past or present depression
- Tendency to somatize
- Belief that serious disease is present and that prognosis is poor
- Secondary gain from 'sick role', including ongoing litigation
- Tendency to view problems in catastrophic fashion.

Examination

General

- The first step should be to gauge whether there are features of systemic ill-health. Does the patient look ill, pale or wasted? Is he febrile? Are there lymph nodes, breast masses, abnormal chest or abdominal signs? (Beware of aortic aneurysms that occasionally present with lumbar pain.)
- Observe the gait. Is there an apparent discrepancy in leg length? Are there non-spinal features that might suggest a spondyloarthropathy (psoriasis, large joint arthritis)?
- Is the observed degree of pain congruent with the history? Does the patient appear depressed?

The spine and legs

Inspection and palpation of the back contributes little to the assessment, but note the following:
- Muscle spasm
- Localized tenderness (crush fracture or metastatic involvement at that level?)
- Kyphosis or scoliosis
- Palpable step in spine
- Hairy patch over sacrum (closed neural tube defect?).

Movements of the cervical and lumbar spine should be assessed in all four directions. A crude measure of lumbar flexion can be made by placing a finger at either end of the lumbar spine and asking the patient to bend forward. If the distance between the fingers increases by 5 cm or more, serious pathology is unlikely. Global restriction of spinal movement should raise thoughts of ankylosing spondylitis.

Restriction of passive straight-leg raising suggests nerve root entrapment on that side. Consider assessing the validity of this finding by sitting the patient forward with his or her legs in front on the couch. Severe root entrapment is unlikely if the legs can be placed at or near 90°.

Assess power and sensation in the legs. The detail required should be determined by the patient's symptoms. Assess perineal sensation and anal tone if there is even a remote suggestion of cauda equina involvement. Absence of reflexes is the firmest sign of root dysfunction at that level.

In examining the patient with back pain, look for the following:
- Is there evidence of systemic ill-health?
- Are there unilateral neurological signs?
- Is there evidence of cauda equina compression?

Approach to investigations and management

Investigations

Investigation is unlikely to be helpful in a patient with typical acute or chronic mechanical low back pain [2]. If anything this may cause iatrogenic harm by revealing incidental radiological changes of doubtful significance, which often reinforce the patient's belief that they have a serious and irreversible problems with their back. Occasionally patients may find negative investigation reassuring.

The presence of unilateral limb symptoms does not usually indicate a need for immediate investigation because most patients with apparent root entrapment settle spontaneously. The decision to investigate should usually be made only if the results of investigation are likely to influence management. The severity of neurological symptoms is important. Severe, disabling, motor deficits (such as foot drop) are less likely to resolve spontaneously and more likely to need intervention than purely pain or sensory disturbance. Progression of neurological features moves the patient into red flag territory and towards urgent assessment. The most useful diagnostic tool in the assessment of unilateral limb symptoms is MRI [3].

In patients with back pain, 'red flag' symptoms require urgent investigation and sometimes, as in the case of cauda equina compression, immediate investigation.

General

In suspected inflammatory (Case B) or neoplastic (Case D) back pain, perform the following tests:
- Blood count
- Renal and liver function
- Calcium, alkaline phosphatase
- Immunoglobulins and electrophoresis of serum and urine
- Blood cultures
- Chest radiograph.

Spinal imaging

Plain radiographs of the lumbar spine and sacroiliac joints are helpful in ankylosing spondylitis, and may reveal patterns of bony destruction suggestive of infective discitis and malignancy. MRI, however, is the imaging technique most likely to establish the diagnosis (Fig. 15). Interventional radiology or surgery may then be required to provide a definitive microbiological or histological diagnosis.

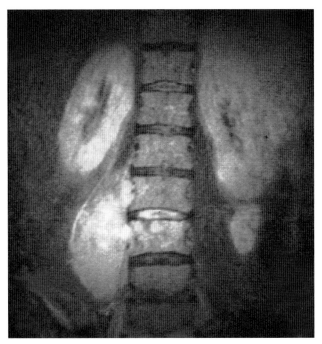

Fig. 15 Coronal MRI from a patient who presented with a 2-week history of back pain and a 1-day history of perineal anaesthesia. The scan shows infiltration of the body of L3 and right psoas muscle. Histological diagnosis: high-grade non-Hodgkin's lymphoma.

Management

Management is determined by the cause.

Mechanical back pain

The following are useful practical measures for patients such as the man in Case A:
- Encourage mobilization
- Simple analgesia
- Graded rehabilitative exercise programme
- Some benefit can be gained from manipulation in acute pain
- Treat depression.

Patients with mechanical back pain should be discouraged from resting and directed towards a long-term rehabilitative approach to their backs. In chronic pain, there may be many barriers to this approach and outcomes may be limited. A firm, sympathetic, but realistic approach is required. Aim to improve function rather than cure chronic pain. Identify patients with acute or recurrent pain at high risk of chronicity for particular attention.

Root entrapment syndromes

Most of these syndromes will settle within weeks, so defer intervention unless a severe motor defect is present. Encourage mobilization. There is probable benefit from epidural corticosteroids. A minority with persistent symptoms will require surgery.

Serious pathology

Treat the underlying cause. Spinal cord compression or cauda equina syndrome require immediate consideration of surgery (Case C).

Management of the patient with back pain

- Mechanical pain: minimal investigation, maximum mobilization
- Unilateral nerve root pain: mobilize, but wait and see
- Red flag features: urgent investigation and management.

See *Emergency medicine*, Section 1.23.
See *Neurology*, Section 1.13.
1 Klippel JH, Dieppe PA (eds). *Rheumatology*, 2nd edn. London: Mosby, 1998. Section 4, Parts 3 and 6.
2 Royal College of General Practitioners. *Clinical Guidelines for the Management of Acute Low Back Pain*. London: Royal College of General Practitioners, 1999.
3 Van Tulder MW. Low back pain and sciatica. In: *Clinical Evidence*, Issue 2. London: BMJ Publishing, 1999: 406–422.

1.18 Acute hot joints

Case histories

Case A

A 73-year-old woman presents with a 24-h history of a painful swollen right knee. She feels generally unwell and her GP found her temperature to be 38.1°C. She has had minor pain and stiffness in both knees for many years.

Case B

A 42-year-old man presents with a hot swollen left elbow. He gives a past history of two attacks of severe pain and redness of the big toes over the last 2 years. He is overweight and drinks 4–5 pints of beer several nights a week.

Case C

A 21-year-old man developed a painful swollen right knee 1 week after returning from holidaying in Spain. Two days later he developed pain and swelling in the left midfoot. He denied any recent episodes of diarrhoea or genitourinary symptoms.

Table 15 Differential diagnosis of acute hot joints.

Frequency of disorder	Examples
Common	Crystal arthritis
	Gout (Case B)
	Pseudogout (Case A)
	Reactive arthritis (Case C)
	Non-gonococcal septic arthritis caused by
	pyogenic bacteria
	Staph. aureus (70%)
	Other Gram-positive cocci (20%)
	Gram-negative bacilli (10%)
Rare	Haemarthrosis
	Other spondyloarthritides
	Other infections
	Gonococcal arthritis (rare in the UK, more
	common in the USA, Australasia)
	Lyme disease
	Palindromic rheumatism
	Monoarticular presentation of rheumatoid arthritis
	Osteonecrosis (especially involving the hip)

Clinical approach

Could this be septic arthritis? This is the primary concern in the assessment of the acute hot joint. Septic arthritis is not the most common cause of an acute monoarthritis (Table 15) but it is the most serious, with potential for severe joint damage and life-threatening septicaemia. If sepsis has been considered and excluded, the main differential diagnosis is between a crystal arthritis and a postinfective reactive arthritis. The history and examination may give pointers towards the correct diagnosis, but sepsis can never be completely excluded on this basis alone. The most important tool in the assessment of the acute hot joint is aspiration of synovial fluid for microscopy and culture.

The hot joint

- The best diagnostic tool is synovial fluid aspiration
- Always consider the possible diagnosis of septic arthritis.

History of the presenting problem

The history of joint swelling is usually straightforward but helps little with the differential diagnosis. A history of trauma may point to haemarthrosis. Rapid onset of pain and systemic malaise can occur in all the common causes, but severe systemic symptoms should increase the suspicion of sepsis. A slow, subacute onset makes pyogenic bacterial sepsis less likely. The differential diagnosis is influenced by age. Crystal arthritis is the most common cause in elderly people, whereas reactive arthritis tends to occur in sexually active young adults. Gout and reactive arthritis are more common in men.

Relevant past history

Consider the diagnoses listed in Table 15—which of these fits the picture best?

Risk factors for sepsis

- Is there a history of penetrating injury (either near the joint or elsewhere), which might have acted as a portal of entry? Don't forget intravenous drug abuse.
- Is there a history of immunosuppression (especially corticosteroid treatment)?

Previous similar episodes

Episodic severe flitting monoarthritis raises particular suspicions of gout, especially if the first metatarsophalangeal joint has been involved. Palindromic rheumatism may produce a similar picture.

Chronic rheumatological disease

A history suggestive of prior osteoarthritis in the hot joint may point to pseudogout. Patients with rheumatoid arthritis have an increased risk of sepsis (independent of treatment, but steroid therapy increases the risk further).

Risk factors for gout

Gout is far more common in men, obese individuals and people who drink heavily. A family history is also common. Diuretics (especially thiazides and furosemide [frusemide]) are a common predisposing factor, especially in elderly people. Gout hardly ever occurs in women except in the context of diuretic usage.

Infection

Is there any evidence of infection that might trigger a reactive arthritis? Rheumatologists reserve the term 'reactive arthritis' for a specific syndrome of acute non-infectious mono- or oligoarthritis, with a predilection for the large joints of the legs, which occurs after bacterial gastrointestinal infection (*Salmonella*, *Shigella*, *Campylobacter* or *Yersinia* spp.) or sexually acquired chlamydial infection. Arthritis can occur alone or together with ocular and mucocutaneous disease, when the label Reiter's syndrome can be used. Ask about recent travel, diarrhoeal illness and genitourinary symptoms such as penile or vaginal discharge.

Taking a sexual history

It may be necessary to take a sexual history, but this should be sensitively handled because patients are usually unaware of any possible link between their painful knee and their sex life. This discussion should therefore be left to the end of the consultation, after the rest of the history and examination have been performed, and the topic should be introduced carefully, with explanation, perhaps as follows:

'I need to ask one or two more questions to try to work out why your knee is giving trouble …'

'There are many reasons why it might be …'

'Some infections can cause the problem …'

'In particular, some genital infections can do this …'

'Are you at risk of any of these …?'

'Have you had any problems in that department?'

'Have you had any discharge or ulceration on your penis/vagina?'

'Have you had sex with any new partners recently?'

(See *General clinical issues*, Section 2.)

Examination

A sick febrile patient should always be considered to have sepsis until proven otherwise. However, sepsis can be present in the patient who initially appears clinically well (especially if elderly or immunosuppressed).

Confirm that the swelling is articular rather than periarticular or subcutaneous. Is an effusion present? Erythema around the joint can occur in gout but should raise a very strong suspicion of sepsis.

Are the other joints normal? Is there evidence of a more widespread acute inflammatory arthropathy? Are there features of a chronic arthritis preceding the acute illness?

Look for features suggestive of reactive arthritis/Reiter's syndrome:

- Conjunctivitis/uveitis
- Scaly rashes on the palms and soles
- Balanitis
- Urethral discharge.

Look for tophi, which can occur on any pressure point.

Approach to investigations and management

Investigations

Joint aspiration

Investigation of a hot joint

Aspiration of synovial fluid is vital for accurate diagnosis. Techniques are not difficult, but if you are not confident ask someone else. On call, these skills are most likely to be found among the orthopaedic team. Do not defer aspiration because you lack this skill (see Section 3.5, pp. 107–108).

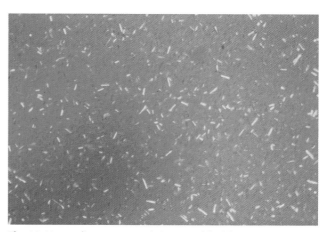

Fig. 16 Monosodium urate crystals in synovial fluid from acute gout observed by polarized light microscopy.

A few drops of fluid are sufficient for microscopy and culture (Fig. 16). The macroscopic appearance of synovial fluid may give some clues:

- Grossly purulent fluid suggests sepsis
- Blood-stained fluid may suggest haemarthrosis but also occurs in pseudogout.

Fluid should be sent urgently for:

- Polarized light microscopy for crystals
- Gram stain for organisms
- Culture.

Only rarely does gout coexist with sepsis (unless there is an ulcerating tophus), although pseudogout can; hence, it may be best to wait 24 h for culture results before concluding that pseudogout is the primary diagnosis.

Other tests

Blood cultures are mandatory when sepsis is suspected.

Other blood tests provide less diagnostic information:

- FBC: the white cell count may be normal in acute sepsis.
- Serum urate is of no value in making a diagnosis of acute gout.
- Inflammatory markers: a measure of the acute phase response is helpful in measuring the subsequent response to therapy.
- Autoantibody testing: hardly ever helpful in this context.
- Clotting screen: should be performed in those with haemarthrosis.
- Radiographs: largely unhelpful, showing evidence of chronic joint disease only.

Management

Immediate management should be:

- Admit to hospital if there is a strong suspicion of sepsis or mobility is severely restricted. If sepsis is unlikely, the patient may be managed as an outpatient with early follow-up.
- Start empirical antibiotic therapy if sepsis is clinically

likely—purulent synovial fluid or organisms on Gram stain. In adults, use high-dose flucloxacillin plus a third-generation cephalosporin initially.
• Antibiotics can be withdrawn if cultures are negative at 24 h. Six weeks is the minimum period of antibiotic treatment for sepsis (usually 2 weeks i.v.).

 Beware prior antibiotic treatment masking the diagnosis of sepsis.

Note the following:
• Orthopaedic assessment is mandatory in sepsis: arthrotomy/joint wash-out may be indicated. Orthopaedic surgeons should deal with suspected sepsis in a prosthetic joint from an early stage.
• NSAIDs may give useful symptom control but avoid them in the presence of renal impairment (often present in this context). Beware of past or current history suggestive of peptic ulceration, reflux or NSAID intolerance.
• Treatment of non-septic arthritides with intra-articular steroids may be indicated. In most patients, do this only after negative culture, although some may be injected at the time of initial assessment (e.g. recurrent gout). If in doubt, wait.
• Consider unusual infections (e.g. TB, fungal) in patients with immunosuppression or a history of foreign travel.
• Avoid weight bearing on a severely inflamed joint, but splintage is not usually necessary. Arrange for early mobilization as inflammation subsides—physiotherapy input will be required.

Do not forget longer-term issues:
• Screening for chlamydial infection in sexually active patients with non-crystal, non-septic arthritis
• Gout prophylaxis
• Gout as a surrogate marker for diabetes, hypertension, hyperlipidaemia.

 See *Infectious diseases*, Sections 1.31, 1.32, 1.33 and 1.34.
1 Joint Working Group of the British Society for Rheumatology and the Research Unit of the Royal College of Physicians. Guidelines and proposed audit protocol for the initial management of an acute hot joint. *J R Coll Physicians Lond* 1992; 26: 83–85.

1.19 Recurrent joint pain and morning stiffness

Case history

A 55-year-old woman presents with polyarticular arthritis. She has had several attacks of pain and swelling affecting the metacarpophalangeal and proximal interphalangeal joints over the past few months, with morning stiffness and fatigue.

Clinical approach

Although rheumatoid arthritis is the most likely diagnosis in a middle-aged woman with small-joint polyarthritis, other possible diagnoses, e.g. systemic lupus or psoriatic arthritis, should not be overlooked.

History of the presenting problem

Severity of joint symptoms

Ask the following if the details do not emerge spontaneously:
• What is the duration, site and character of the pain?
• How fast did it come on? The majority of cases of rheumatoid arthritis develop insidiously over weeks or months.
• How much is movement limited? What functions are difficult to perform? Ask about feeding, washing, combing the hair and walking.
• Are there any features suggestive of inflammation? Early morning stiffness that improves as the day goes on is a non-specific feature of inflammatory disease. Tiredness, lethargy and feeling generally unwell are features of active disease.
• What is the pattern of joint involvement? Is it monoarticular, oligoarticular or polyarticular? Additive or migratory? Additive polyarticular symmetrical presentation is typical of rheumatoid arthritis.

 Different patterns of onset of rheumatoid arthritis

• Acute monoarthritis (see Section 1.18, pp. 36–39)
• Acute polyarthritis
• Subacute, insidious polyarthritis
• Polymyalgic presentation, particularly in elderly people; important to differentiate from polymyalgia rheumatica (see Section 2.5.1, pp. 88–89).

Relevant past history

Direct questioning is vital because it may reveal important extra-articular symptoms which are helpful in the differential diagnosis:
• Skin rash (psoriasis, butterfly rash and photosensitivity)
• Raynaud's phenomenon
• Red eyes
• Urethritis and dysentery.

Consider psoriatic arthritis
- Distal interphalangeal joints commonly involved
- Characteristic psoriatic nail changes
- Joint involvement typically asymmetrical
- Sausage-shaped finger characteristic (dactylitis)
- High ESR and CRP with negative rheumatoid factor
- Sacroiliac (SI) joint involvement.

Consider SLE
- Younger age group
- Jaccoud-type arthropathy
- No radiological bone erosions
- High ESR but normal CRP
- ANA positive in 99–100% of cases
- Rheumatoid factor variable but usually negative
- Photosensitivity and renal impairment.

Examination

Avoid shaking hands with a patient with active arthritis of the hands, or do so very gently!

General

Look for systemic features associated with active rheumatoid arthritis: pallor, lymphadenopathy, fever and weight loss.

In the skin look for the following:
- Rheumatoid nodules: seen in 25% of cases and correlates with rheumatoid factor seropositivity and rapidly progressive disease. Commonly found at pressure points such as the elbows, sacrum and occiput.
- Palmar erythema and cutaneous vasculitis.

Full assessment of the other systems is essential in all cases with polyarticular presentation (see Section 2.3.3, pp. 72–74).

Severity of arthritis

Each joint is assessed fully using the following format: look, feel, move.

Look

Look for the following:
- Joint deformity
- Swelling of the joints
- Skin redness (acute infection or inflammation), tophi, psoriatic plaques and rheumatoid nodules
- Muscle bulk, for any evidence of wasting in the main muscle groups that move the affected joint.

Feel

Feel for the following:
- Warmth by comparing the temperature of the skin overlying the affected joint with that of the normal contralateral side.
- Tenderness by very gentle pressure over the joint line (e.g. ball of the foot for metatarsophalangeal [MTP] synovitis)
- Nature of the swelling—usually soft synovial tissue in rheumatoid arthritis and bony in osteoarthritis.

Move

Painful limitation of motion usually indicates active synovitis. Patients often complain of poor hand grip and inability to open doors or cut bread.

In rheumatoid arthritis, the small joints of the hands and feet are most commonly involved, namely:
- Proximal interphalangeal joints (PIPs)
- Metacarpophalangeal joints (MCPs)
- Metatarsophalangeal joints (MTPs).

The distribution of joint involvement is bilateral and symmetrical.

Locomotor assessment

Use the acronym 'GALS' as an *aide-mémoire* for overall assessment of the locomotor system:
- G: gait
- A: arm
- L: leg
- S: spine.

Consider osteoarthritis (generalized nodal osteoarthritis)
- Hands are commonly affected with Heberden's and Bouchard's nodes
- Early morning stiffness for <30 min
- Symptoms are worse after exercise
- ESR and CRP are usually normal
- Negative rheumatoid factor
- Characteristic radiological changes. Marginal erosions are not a feature of osteoarthritis.

Remember that acute synovitis in early rheumatoid arthritis is associated with very little fixed joint deformity and no extra-articular features. This contrasts with the deforming arthritis that is characteristic of chronic disease (Fig. 17).

Approach to investigations and management

Investigations

The diagnosis of rheumatoid arthritis is based on a collection of features rather than a specific pathognomonic abnormality.

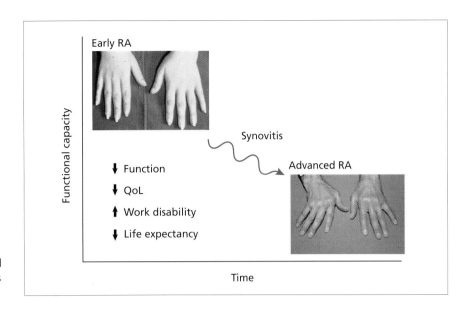

Fig. 17 Deforming arthropathy in rheumatoid arthritis. (Courtesy of Professor P Emery, Leeds General Infirmary.)

Blood tests

Check the following:
- FBC: may show anaemia of chronic disease.
- Inflammatory markers: ESR and CRP are expected to be high in inflammatory arthritis and normal in osteoarthritis.
- Rheumatoid factor: positive in 70% of cases of rheumatoid arthritis and usually negative in osteoarthritis. Seronegative arthropathies are rheumatoid factor negative by definition.
- Renal and liver function tests: likely to be normal, but important to establish pretreatment baseline.
- Other immunological tests, e.g. ANA, may be indicated in some cases (see Sections 1.11, pp. 22–24 and 3.2, pp. 98–101).

Radiographs

Radiological changes in rheumatoid arthritis are usually seen in the hands, wrists and feet, although radiographs may be normal in early disease. Radiographs of other clinically involved joints are recommended. Serial radiographs of the affected joints provide a useful clue to disease progression and response to treatment (see Sections 2.3.3, p. 74 and 3.4, pp. 104–105).

Arthrocentesis

Examination of synovial fluid may be useful in selected cases to differentiate rheumatoid arthritis from non-inflammatory arthritis and crystal arthritis (see Section 3.5, pp. 107–108).

Management

The principles of management are based on the following [1, 2]:

- Relief of symptoms (simple analgesia and NSAIDs and intra-articular steroids)
- Prevention of structural damage and deformity (disease-modifying antirheumatic drugs, immunotherapy, surgery)
- Preservation of function (physiotherapy, occupational therapy)
- Maintenance of the patient's normal lifestyle (occupational therapy and social support).

See *Medicine for the elderly*, Section 1.5.
1 Van Gestel AM, Stucki G. Evaluation of established rheumatoid arthritis. *Best Practice Res Clin Rheumatol* 1999; 13: 629–644.
2 Emery P, Marzo H, Proudman S. Management of patients with newly diagnosed rheumatoid arthritis. *Rheumatology (Oxford)* 1999; 38(suppl 2): 27–31.

1.20 Foot drop and weight loss

Case history

A 60-year-old man with a 10-year history of erosive seropositive nodular rheumatoid arthritis is referred to hospital with a recent left foot drop and progressive weight loss.

Clinical approach

The onset of foot drop in a patient with seropositive rheumatoid arthritis is very suggestive of systemic rheumatoid vasculitis [1]. Although many of the features of systemic rheumatoid vasculitis may also occur in other systemic vasculitides such as polyarteritis nodosa (PAN) (Table 16), in practice there is little difficulty in differentiating between the two.

Feature	SRV	PAN
Joints	Almost always occurs on a background of seropositive, nodular rheumatoid arthritis	Arthralgia in 50% Frank non-deforming arthritis in 20%
Skin, purpura, digital infarcts	+	+
Mononeuritis multiplex	+	+
Glomerulonephritis	<5%	Rare in classic PAN
Angiography	Not useful	Diagnostically useful investigation revealing aneurysms of visceral arteries
Hepatitis B surface antigen	No association	Positive in 20%
Complement (C3, C4)	Normal or ↓	Normal or ↓
ANCA	p-ANCA in 10–20%	Negative in classic PAN

Table 16 Comparison of systemic rheumatoid vasculitis (SRV) and polyarteritis nodosa (PAN).

p-ANCA, antineutrophil cytoplasmic antibody.

History of the presenting problem

As systemic rheumatoid vasculitis occurs on a background of chronic rheumatoid arthritis, your questions should be directed towards the following:
• Clarifying the behaviour of the patient's rheumatoid arthritis with particular reference to extra-articular disease
• Assessing the severity of the foot drop
• Determining what, if anything, precipitated this episode. Could it have been infection or drugs?

Systemic rheumatoid vasculitis

At presentation, non-specific systemic features such as weight loss will often predominate without specific vasculitic features. Consequently, the clinical picture may be reminiscent of malignancy, particularly in men who smoke.

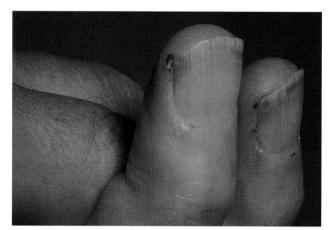

Fig. 18 Nail-fold digital infarcts in rheumatoid vasculitis. (With permission from *Arthritis and Rheumatism in Practice*, Merck, Gower Medical Publishing.)

Consider systemic rheumatoid vasculitis in rheumatoid arthritis in the presence of:
• persistent fever, fatigue and unexplained weight loss (95%)
• painful red eye—scleritis, 'corneal melt' syndrome
• nail-fold infarcts, splinter haemorrhages, chronic leg and sacral ulcers, and digital gangrene (Figs 18–20)
• small intracutaneous nodules
• mononeuritis multiplex (50%)
• glomerulonephritis (<5%).
Percentages refer to the frequency of a particular feature in systemic rheumatoid vasculitis.

Examination

See Section 1.19, p. 40, and in addition perform a detailed neurological examination looking for evidence of mononeuritis multiplex.

Synovitis may be surprisingly inactive in systemic rheumatoid vasculitis—a diagnostic pitfall for the unwary.

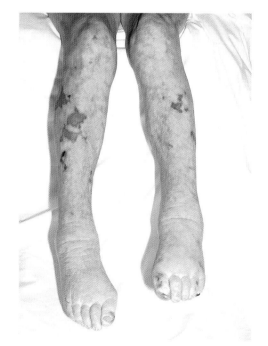

Fig. 19 Vasculitic skin rash in rheumatoid arthritis.

Approach to investigations and management

Investigations

Investigation should be aimed at assessing the severity of rheumatoid arthritis and obtaining histological evidence of vasculitis. Those tests indicated in Section 1.19, p. 41 will be required, taking particular note of the following (some of which are additional):

• Acute phase indices: both CRP and ESR are invariably raised with active disease.

• Rheumatoid factor: likely to be positive in patients with systemic rheumatoid vasculitis but does not correlate with severity of vasculitis.

• Dipstix urine for proteinuria and haematuria: if positive, microscope for red cell casts. Check renal function. Could this man have rheumatoid renal vasculitis, which is rare but possible?

• Tissue biopsy: obtain histological evidence of vasculitis wherever possible. Sural nerve biopsy can be useful in the diagnosis of mononeuritis multiplex if you have an experienced biopsier and skilled neuropathologist. Alternatively, biopsying tender muscle is often informative.

• Electrophysiological studies: document extent and type of neuropathy.

Management

Aim to treat vasculitis and optimize control of rheumatoid arthritis:

• Isolated cutaneous vasculitis confined to the nail folds does not warrant cytotoxic therapy, but severe rheumatoid vasculitis invariably requires immunosuppressive therapy with steroids and cyclophosphamide

• Ensure that his rheumatoid arthritis is itself optimally controlled with appropriate disease-modifying antirheumatic drug therapy (DMARD).

See *Nephrology*, Sections 1.4, 1.9 and 2.7.5.
1 Vollertson RS, Conn DL. Vasculitis associated with rheumatoid arthritis. *Rheum Disease Clin North Am* 1990; 16: 445–461.

1.21 Fever, myalgia, arthralgia and elevated acute phase indices

---

Case history

A 50-year-old man presents with a 4-month history of episodic pyrexia, myalgia, arthralgia and loss of weight. Further questioning reveals testicular pain and a recent history of postprandial abdominal pain. The results of initial investigations are as follows:

• Neutrophilia (11×10^9/L)
• ESR 110 mm/h, CRP 80 mg/L
• ANA negative
• ANCA negative
• Rheumatoid factor (RF) negative
• Serum immunoglobulins and complement C3 and C4 levels normal
• Repeated blood cultures have produced no growth
• Chest radiography and echocardiography are normal, as are CT scans of the chest, abdomen and pelvis.

Clinical approach

Persistent episodic fever, systemic symptoms and a marked acute phase response in a middle-aged patient may be caused by a wide range of disorders, all of which must be considered (Table 17). Of the vasculitides, Wegener's granulomatosis and microscopic polyangiitis are rendered unlikely (but not excluded) by the negative ANCA. The negative ANA effectively excludes lupus. Polyarteritis nodosa remains a diagnostic possibility (see Table 16) and is compatible with the clinical presentation and results of initial investigations.

 Polyarteritis nodosa

American College of Rheumatology criteria for the classification of polyarteritis nodosa [1] are given below. PAN should be considered as a diagnosis if a patient has at least three of these criteria:

• Weight loss
• Livedo reticularis
• Testicular pain or tenderness
• Myalgia
• Mononeuropathy or polyneuropathy
• Diastolic BP >90 mmHg
• Renal impairment
• Hepatitis B antigenaemia (particularly in Oriental patients with a high background prevalence of hepatitis B)
• Arteriographic abnormality
• Biopsy of small or medium-sized artery containing polymorphs.

History of the presenting problem

Polyarteritis nodosa

Clarify the nature of the following:
• Pyrexia and systemic symptoms
• Abdominal pain: recurrent postprandial central abdominal pain may indicate critical bowel ischaemia ('mesenteric claudication').

Ask about the following:
• Has he had a skin rash and, if so, is this compatible with cutaneous vasculitis?

Type of disorder	Comment
Infection	Bacterial
	Subacute bacterial endocarditis and TB are the most likely
	Consider liver abscess
	Viral
	Infection with EBV and CMV can be persistent
	Other
	Consider malaria in anyone who might have been exposed
	Consider wider differential in anyone who has been to the tropics
	or who is immunosuppressed for any reason
Inflammatory disorders	Autoimmune rheumatic disorders
	Lupus and lupus overlap disorders
	Adult-onset Still's disease
	Rheumatoid arthritis
	Other
	Sarcoidosis
	Vasculitis: microscopic polyangiitis, Wegener's granulomatosis,
	polyarteritis nodosa (PAN)
	Drug fever
Malignancies	Haematological—lymphoma
	Renal
Other	A very few cases will be factitious

Table 17 Differential diagnosis of persistent fever (>2 weeks), systemic symptoms and a marked acute phase response in an adult who is not immunosuppressed.

CMV, cytomegalovirus; EBV, Epstein–Barr virus.

- Has he had numbness, paraesthesiae or muscle weakness that might indicate mononeuritis multiplex?
- Exposure to recreational drugs, particularly in a younger patient, e.g. cocaine-induced vasculitis, may mimic PAN.

Other diagnoses

Consider the diagnostic possibilities listed in Table 17 when taking the history: are there any leads to one or other of these conditions? Haematuria might indicate hypernephroma. Dental extraction 4 months previously might have led to endocarditis, masked by two courses of antibiotics given for fever, etc.

Relevant past history

Is there a history of TB exposure, cardiac abnormality, risk factor for endocarditis, travel abroad, blood transfusion, known malignancy? Ask about hepatitis B infection because hepatitis B surface antigenaemia is a feature of 10–20% of cases of PAN [2] and may affect management (see below).

Examination

The patient will probably have been examined many times, but don't rely on this and perform a thorough examination yourself. Look for the following in particular,

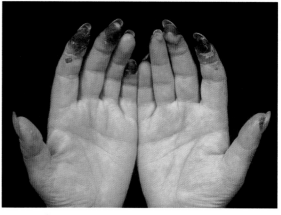

Fig. 20 Digital gangrene in polyarteritis nodosa (PAN).

although many of the possibilities (e.g. organomegaly) will already have been excluded by investigation:
- General: note temperature and look for pallor and lymphadenopathy.
- Skin: examine closely for livedo reticularis, digital gangrene (Fig. 20) and palpable purpura (Fig. 21).
- Cardiovascular: BP is often elevated in PAN, but is clearly not specific for this! Are there any cardiac murmurs? (How good was the echocardiogram?)
- Abdomen: is there any tenderness in view of the possibility of small bowel ischaemia? Is there hepatosplenomegaly, perhaps a pointer towards lymphoma? Is either kidney palpable, perhaps as a result of hypernephroma?

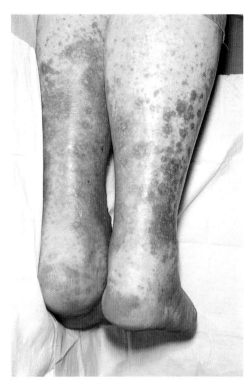

Fig. 21 Necrotic purpuric rash in PAN.

• Testicles: this man has testicular pain—orchitis is a characteristic feature of PAN (see above).
• Neurological: is there mononeuritis multiplex?

Approach to investigations and management

Investigations

When dealing with any patient who has been extensively investigated, but in whom no clear diagnosis has been made, it is vital to review all of the available tests. Is the CT scan really normal? Take it along to an expert, give them a detailed history and ask for their opinion. In this case, thorough review revealed no 'surprises', and PAN seemed the most likely diagnosis on clinical grounds.

Classic PAN is rare in comparison to Wegener's granulomatosis and microscopic polyangiitis (MPA). The following investigations are useful in clarifying the diagnosis of PAN:
• FBC: neutrophilia is expected, occasionally eosinophilia
• Check acute phase markers: both CRP and ESR will be elevated and reflect disease activity
• Hepatitis B status
• Visceral angiography for evidence of aneurysms and arterial occlusion
• Tissue biopsy: consider sural nerve biopsy in patients with neuropathy and skin biopsy in patients with cutaneous features. Alternatively a 'blind' muscle biopsy is often informative.

PAN versus MPA

Differentiating PAN from MPA in a patient with systemic vasculitis:
• Glomerulonephritis
• ANCA positivity
• Normal visceral angiography.
} favours MPA rather than PAN

Management

See Section 2.5.3, p. 92.

See *Nephrology*, Sections 1.9, 2.7.5 and 2.7.6.
1 Lightfoot RW Jr, Michel BA, Block DA *et al.* The American College of Rheumatology 1990 criteria for the classification of polyarteritis nodosa. *Arthritis Rheum* 1990; 33: 1068–1073.
2 Guillevin L, Lhote F, Cohen P *et al.* Polyarteritis nodosa related to Hepatitis B virus—a prospective study with longterm observation of 41 patients. *Medicine (Baltimore)* 1995; 74: 238–253.

1.22 Non-rheumatoid pain and stiffness

Case history

A 55-year-old woman is referred with suspected rheumatoid arthritis. She gives a 3-year history of pain and stiffness in her hands, knees, neck and low back, and a 1-year history of painful swelling in the hands. Examination shows Heberden's nodes in many distal interphalangeal joints, moderate restriction of the neck and painful crepitus in the knees.

Clinical approach

Aim for a reliable differentiation of inflammatory synovitis from degenerative joint disease. This woman seems to have got the latter: you need to determine the pattern of osteoarthritis, consider (briefly) whether any rare underlying cause may be present, and then address symptom control and optimization of function.

History of the presenting problem

Osteoarthritis may be hard to differentiate from inflammatory arthritis by history alone. In general, degenerative joint disease will:
• have a longer, less progressive history
• be associated with only brief stiffness after inactivity (rather than prolonged early morning stiffness)

45

- worsen with activity
- not be associated with joint swelling, except in the fingers
- tend to be associated with pain in the neck and low back.

However, none of these is a totally reliable discriminator in itself.

Relevant past history

Ask about family history (often strong in generalized nodal osteoarthritis) and previous trauma (important predisposing factor in single joints). Occupation may be relevant.

 History of osteoarthritis, type 2 diabetes and liver disease may point to haemochromatosis.

Examination

 Follow the clinical algorithm: look, feel, move.

The distribution of polyarticular joint disease tells you more about the diagnosis than anything else:
- Swelling of the distal interphalangeal joints really only occurs in nodal osteoarthritis (Fig. 22) and one of the forms of psoriatic arthritis, which is usually easily distinguished by nail involvement.
- Involvement of the base of the thumb (the first carpometacarpal joint) is also pathognomonic of nodal osteoarthritis, giving the thumb base a characteristically square appearance.

The most reliable way of assessing the pathology underlying swelling of a single joint is by palpation. In osteoarthritic joints, this reveals that the apparent joint swelling is the result of bony osteophyte growth, by contrast to the boggy swollen soft tissues of the synovitic joint. The joint is usually cool. Effusions may be apparent, but usually only in large joints such as the knee. Movement of any arthritic joint is likely to be painful and restricted, although osteoarthritic joints also often have palpable (and sometimes audible) creaking and scraping, known as crepitus.

Be alert to an unusual pattern of osteoarthritis affecting the metacarpophalangeal joints, usually also with some involvement of the lower-limb large joints. This is associated with calcium pyrophosphate deposition in the affected joints and is most importantly associated with hereditary haemochromatosis.

 Recognizing an osteoarthritic joint
- Distribution: distal interphalangeal (DIP) joints and base of thumb
- Cool, bony swelling
- Restricted movement with crepitus.

Approach to investigations and management

Investigations

Radiological

Radiographs in osteoarthritis reveal the following (Fig. 23):
- Loss of joint space
- Sclerotic bone either side of the joint
- Bony spurs (osteophytes) at the joint margin.
 Less frequently, radiographs may reveal the following:
- Cystic changes in subchondral bone
- Chondrocalcinosis (suggesting calcium pyrophosphate deposition).

Other tests

Synovial fluid aspiration (see Section 3.5, pp. 107–108) is mandatory if there is any suggestion of acute inflammation

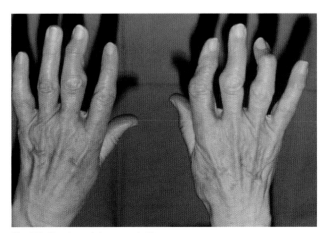

Fig. 22 Classic nodal osteoarthritis.

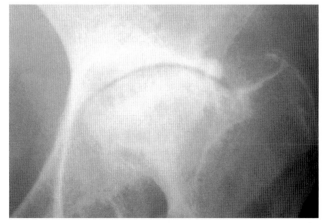

Fig. 23 Radiograph showing severe osteoarthritis of the hip with loss of joint space, subchondral sclerosis and osteophyte formation. (Courtesy of Dr M Pattrick.)

within the joint because osteoarthritic joints have an increased risk of septic arthritis. Even if sepsis is not likely, aspiration may be helpful diagnostically. Fluid from an osteoarthritic joint is typically clear (as it contains no inflammatory cells) and viscous.

Blood tests may be helpful in selected cases. Normal acute inflammatory markers (ESR and CRP) help to rule out an inflammatory arthritis. Ferritin, serum iron and iron binding should be measured if haemochromatosis (see *Endocrinology*, Sections 1.5 and 2.5.3) is suspected.

Management

- The medical management of osteoarthritis is aimed at reducing pain and maximizing function
- This woman will require explanation that her arthritis is not the result of 'rheumatoid'.

Analgesics and NSAIDs (if analgesics fail) are the main drug treatments for osteoarthritis. Intra-articular injections of corticosteroids may offer some short-term improvement in symptoms. The role of intra-articular hyaluronan is similar, but this is expensive and has no clear advantage over corticosteroids. The key factor in maintaining function is maximizing muscle strength around the affected joint(s). Advice on specific muscle-strengthening exercises is required and this should be coupled with general exercises to improve overall fitness.

More severely affected joints may require splintage and modifications of function. Referral to an occupational therapist is likely to be helpful. Surgery should be considered when pain disrupts activity and intrudes on rest.

Brandt KD. *Rheum Dis Clinics North Am* 1999; 25: 257–481. Entire issue devoted to osteoarthritis, covering pathogenesis, investigation and treatment.

1.23 A crush fracture

Case history

A 65-year-old woman develops severe lumbar and right flank pain while gardening. She is admitted to a surgical ward with suspected renal colic, but investigation of her urinary tract is normal. A plain radiograph subsequently shows a crush fracture of T12.

Clinical approach

The most likely cause of a vertebral crush fracture in this woman is osteoporosis, but trauma (not likely to be relevant in this case) and local vertebral pathology (especially secondary tumours or myeloma) should be considered. The most common sites for osteoporotic vertebral fractures are mid-dorsal and the thoracolumbar junction, giving potential for confusion with other causes of chest and flank pain.

The important considerations in osteoporosis are:
- Cause (postmenopausal, corticosteroid induced, myeloma, etc.)
- Severity (predictive of risk of further fractures).

The risk of osteoporotic fracture is influenced heavily by the risk of falling. This risk should be assessed and treatable causes addressed (see *Medicine for the elderly*, Sections 1.1 and 2.3).

History of the presenting problem

Osteoporotic fracture

The diagnosis of possible osteoporotic fracture will almost certainly have been made before referral to you, but the condition should be considered in spinal pain with the following characteristics:
- Sudden onset
- Provoked by movement
- Ameliorated by rest
- Present especially in postmenopausal women and others at increased risk of osteoporosis
- Nerve root irritation or entrapment, which may produce referred pain or paraesthesia with dermatomal distribution.

Other causes of the fracture

Are there any clues to a malignant process? Think about the possibilities as you take the history. Has the woman had any of the following symptoms:
- Felt unwell or lost weight recently?
- Had any trouble with her breathing or coughed anything up? This might indicate respiratory pathology (lung cancer?) or anaemia (gastrointestinal bleeding, bone marrow secondaries or myeloma?) in this context.
- Been troubled by indigestion or change in her bowels? (Gastrointestinal malignancy?)
- Had bone pain elsewhere? (Secondaries or myeloma?)

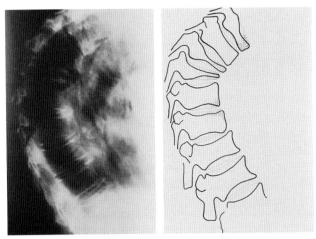

Fig. 24 Multiple osteoporotic fractures in the thoracic spine. (Courtesy of Dr M Pattrick.)

Relevant past history

Osteoporosis

History of femoral neck fracture, Colles' fracture or clinical or radiological evidence of previous vertebral fracture (Fig. 24) are the best surrogate markers of severity of bone loss and future fracture risk.

Causes of osteoporosis

You should ask about the following:
• Menstrual history: at the age of 65 years she will certainly be postmenopausal, but what was her age at menopause, has she had a hysterectomy/oophorectomy or has she had prolonged amenorrhoea at any time, e.g. anorexia nervosa?
• Steroid treatment: risk depends on the dose and duration of treatment.
• Frequency of exercise.
• Dietary history: in particular, does she have an adequate calcium intake?
• Family history.

Risk of falls

Ask about the following:
• Previous falls
• Pre-existing neurological or locomotor disease
• Postural dizziness
• Alcohol use
• Use of psychotropic drugs.

Other causes of vertebral fracture

Has she got a history of malignancy or 'problems with the blood'?

Examination

General

Does the patient look as though she might have malignancy? Your surgical colleagues may have examined the woman thoroughly, but they may not have, so take particular care to look for the following:
• Weight loss, cachexia
• Pallor
• Lymphadenopathy
• A breast lump
• Abnormal chest, abdominal or rectal signs.
  Could the patient have a secondary cause for osteoporosis? Is there evidence to suggest thyrotoxicosis, hypogonadism (in a man) or Cushing's disease?

The spine

The level of the vertebral fracture may be marked by a palpable step. Look for diffuse dorsal kyphosis as a marker of long-standing severe bone loss.

Risk of falling

Look for the following:
• Visible unsteadiness/frailty
• Neurological signs
• Postural drop in blood pressure.

Approach to investigations and management

Investigations

These will obviously be dictated by the findings on history and examination.

Consideration of secondary causes

Need varies, depending on the patient's age, other risk factors, ill-health and clinical suspicion. The following tests should be considered:
• FBC
• Renal and liver function
• Bone biochemistry (raised alkaline phosphatase may suggest osteomalacia or secondaries; hypercalcaemia may suggest malignancy, especially myeloma)
• Immunoglobulins and serum and urine electrophoresis (to exclude myeloma in elderly people)
• Thyroid function
• Testosterone in males
• Investigations for Cushing's syndrome (*Endocrinology*, Section 2.1.1).

Diagnosis of osteoporosis

The gold standard for diagnosis and planning of treatment is bone densitometry at two sites (usually hip and lumbar spine). The presence of a fracture consistent with osteoporosis in the presence of risk factors is often enough to make the diagnosis. Histology is rarely useful and even more rarely obtained.

Management

Pain may be severe and require opiates. Consider supplementary approaches such as TENS (transcutaneous electrical nerve stimulation) machines and epidural analgesia. Immobility will increase the risk of bronchopneumonia and venous thromboembolism (consider prophylactic heparin). Manage secondary causes as identified. Most symptomatic osteoporosis will be postmenopausal and managed by the following:
• Lifestyle modification
• Optimization of calcium intake
• Oestrogen replacement and/or bisphosphonates.

See Section 1.17, pp. 33–36.
See *Pain relief and palliative care*, Section 2.1.
See *Medicine for the elderly*, Sections 1.1, 2.3, 2.8 and 2.11.
See *Haematology*, Sections 1.15 and 2.2.
See *Endocrinology*, Section 2.5.
Klippel JH, Dieppe PA (eds) *Rheumatology*, 2nd edn. London: Mosby, 1998. Section 8, parts 36–38, part 43.
Royal College of Physicians of London. *Osteoporosis: Clinical guidelines for prevention and treatment*. London: Royal College of Physicians of London, 1999.

1.24 Widespread pain

Case history

A 38-year-old woman is referred with a 4-year history of widespread musculoskeletal pain and profound fatigue. She feels that she is slowly becoming weaker and now spends much of the day in bed or in a chair. As a consequence she is heavily dependent on her family. The referral has been prompted by her request for a wheelchair. She describes herself as 'unhappy and unwell'.

She presents as sad, withdrawn and angry. Examination demonstrates very widespread muscular tenderness, and she often winces when touched. However, no abnormal neurological signs can be elicited and joint movements are full, although painful.

Clinical approach

Widespread pain and fatigue have many causes. The case description given here points strongly towards the syndrome known as fibromyalgia, but diagnostic thoughts should be cast wider than this, particularly if 'red flag' features are present.

Red flag features in widespread pain

• Onset age >50 years
• Recent onset, progressive history
• Weight loss
• Previous history of malignancy or immunosuppression
• Focal versus diffuse pain
• Fever
• Any abnormal physical signs other than tenderness
• Abnormal blood tests.

The fibromyalgia syndrome is common and yet diagnostically slippery. Anyone who has worked in a rheumatology clinic will recognize the case scenario described. However, attempts to understand the nature of the disorder within the conventional framework of physical musculoskeletal disease lead to little more than the Cheshire cat's smile. Detailed study has revealed no convincing evidence of musculoskeletal pathology, although the syndrome may arise on a background of definite rheumatic disease (e.g. rheumatoid arthritis, spinal pain). There is considerable overlap with other so-called functional syndromes, particularly the chronic fatigue syndrome, and also a very high prevalence of psychiatric disorders, particularly depression.

Fibromyalgia is best considered as a disorder of bodily perception, in which pain is perceived centrally in the absence of any peripheral cause. This is often intertwined with a tendency to somatize, or express psychological distress in physical terms. Various factors seem to perpetuate the syndrome including the following:
• Sleep disturbance
• A tendency to cope with pain and fatigue by withdrawal and rest
• Consequent profound loss of physical fitness
• Depression.

All of these factors can, to some extent, be addressed. Patients with this clinical picture have a high level of disability, and the cumulative impact of fibromyalgia is greater than that of rheumatoid arthritis. It is not acceptable to simply document the lack of severe physical disease in these patients and then discharge them. They deserve a constructive and positive approach to diagnosis and management.

History of the presenting problem

It seems very likely that this woman has fibromyalgia, but

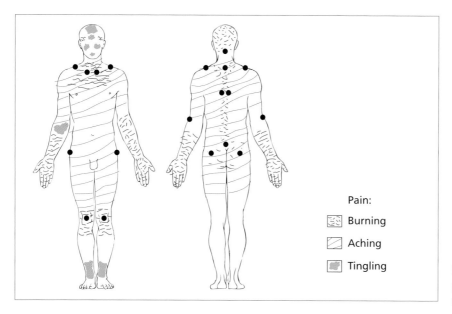

Pain:

Burning

Aching

Tingling

Fig. 25 Pain diagram showing classic tender points (full circles) in fibromyalgia plus patient's own illustration of site and nature of pain.

it would be wrong to assume this immediately, without the benefit of a full systems enquiry. Are any red flag features present?

Fibromyalgia

Document the pattern of pain and its progression over time. Pain in fibromyalgia is very widespread but usually predominantly axial rather than peripheral, typically inexorable but rarely progressive (Fig. 25).

Ask about fatigue. Is this localized muscle weakness (raising suspicions of neurological disease) or a more generalized feeling of tiredness or lack of energy ('tired all the time')? This is often associated with other cognitive symptoms such as difficulty concentrating and a feeling of 'muzzy-headedness'. Other neurological symptoms may be present, particularly flitting paraesthesia.

Gain a picture of the patient's degree of disability and the impact on her life. What is the patient's current exercise capacity? Ask about sleep patterns and sleep disturbance. Is sleep refreshing? Is there a history of other functional syndromes?

Is there evidence of depression currently? Note that other cognitive symptoms may occur, and are often associated with depression. Is there evidence of previous psychiatric illness? Here again, examination of the case notes may be revealing.

> Review of the case notes or discussion with the general practitioner may be particularly helpful. Look for the following:
> - Irritable bowel syndrome
> - Chronic fatigue syndrome/myalgic encephalopathy (ME)
> - Unexplained breathlessness or chest pain
> - Unexplained gynaecological symptoms
> - Unexplained headache or dizziness
> - Multiple 'allergies' in the absence of objective evidence.

Examination

> Most patients with fibromyalgia will give an immediate impression of distress and depression. This is, in itself, striking and significant. The psychological state of patients with most illnesses will depend heavily on their personality and coping strategies. The patient with rheumatoid disease can be cheerful, stoical, anxious or depressed, but the patient with fibromyalgia will invariably be weary and sad. Despite this unhappiness the patient usually appears physically well.

A full general examination is required. The following are typical findings in fibromyalgia:
- Widespread tenderness, with a tendency to wince and withdraw when touched, especially at certain 'trigger points' (see Fig. 25).
- Other physical signs are striking by their absence.
- Joint movement is usually full with gentle encouragement.
- Common rheumatological conditions (e.g. spinal pain, osteoarthritis) will, of course, often also be present in the patient with fibromyalgia.
- Note that any positive neurological signs should cause you to hesitate before applying the label of fibromyalgia.

> Fibromyalgia is a syndrome of symptoms, not signs. If there are any positive physical signs other than tenderness, reconsider the diagnosis.

Approach to investigations and management

Investigations

This requires a balance between the need to exclude serious pathology and the harm that can be done by over-investigation. Patients with fibromyalgia (and other functional syndromes) will often have undergone repeated episodes of negative investigation. This process strongly reinforces the belief that the symptoms have a serious physical cause, which would be identified if only the right tests were performed. However, as further negative investigations are performed, patients come to feel that the doctor does not believe that their symptoms are real ('he thinks it's all in my mind'). The doctor–patient relationship deteriorates, and the patient may move on to repeat the process elsewhere.

The need for investigation should be driven by the degree of clinical suspicion that the diagnosis is not fibromyalgia. Pay attention to the red flag features listed above. Unfortunately, investigation is often driven more by insecurity and lack of experience, leading to a fear of 'missing something'. It is also important that the rationale for investigation be explained to the patient. If you feel that the results are likely to be negative, say so and explain why. A minimalist approach to investigation might include the following:

- FBC
- Renal, bone and liver biochemistry, blood glucose
- Creatinine kinase
- Thyroid function
- Acute phase markers: CRP, ESR
- Myeloma screen in patients >50 years
- Antinuclear antibodies
- Chest radiograph, especially in smokers.

Management

Is the patient likely be helped by the label of fibromyalgia? This is difficult to answer.

Argument against fibromyalgia

Placing a simple diagnostic label on a patient whose problems are at least partly the result of a tendency to express psychological distress in physical terms may serve only to perpetuate the patient's belief that the problems have an external physical cause. This may further divert attention from the real problems.

Argument for fibromyalgia

The diagnostic label can be used constructively to convince patients that their symptoms do fall into a recognized pattern, and to provide a framework for management. This framework can then be used to discuss the relationship between the physical symptoms and depression and other psychological factors. This is often a difficult area, with the potential for breakdown in communication unless tactfully handled.

It is often easier for the patient to accept that further investigation is unlikely to be helpful if it is felt that a diagnosis has been achieved.

How you can help

Patients with a long history and a high degree of disability have a very poor prognosis, and it is hard to improve their management without a diagnostic framework. Involvement of pain management services and liaison psychiatry may be useful. Issues of the sick role, secondary gain and involvement of the family and carers may also need to be addressed. In practice, management of these patients can and should proceed in much the same way, regardless of use of a diagnostic label.

In dealing with patients with fibromyalgia, the following should be the central principles:
- Do not organize more and more investigations
- Give a view of treatment as a process of rehabilitation, in which the patient plays an active part
- Be realistic about the prognosis
- Suggest a graded aerobic exercise programme, aiming to improve overall fitness
- Treat sleep disturbance, usually with low-dose tricyclic antidepressants
- Use analgesics if helpful, but withdraw if they are not
- Consider secondary gain
- Treat depression, and consider psychiatric assessment
- Consider referral for cognitive behaviour therapy, which is particularly useful in countering the negative ideas that most patients have about their illness.

See *General clinical issues*, Section 3.
See *Psychiatry*, Section 1.6.
Leventhal LJ. Management of fibromyalgia. *Ann Intern Med* 1999; 131: 850–858.
Wessely S, Nimnuan C, Sharpe M. Functional somatic syndromes: one or many? *Lancet* 1999; 354: 936–939.

1.25 Fever and absent upper limb pulses

Case history

A 28-year-old Chinese woman is referred with an 18-month history of general ill-health, episodic low-grade fever and absent radial pulses.

Disorder	Comments
Takayasu's arteritis	See text
Giant cell arteritis	May be difficult to differentiate in women >40 years [2]
	Oriental background, subclavian and renal artery involvement favour Takayasu's arteritis
Polyarteritis nodosa	Multi-system involvement, aneurysms of visceral/renal circulation (see Section 1.21, pp. 43–45)
Connective tissue disorders (SLE, rheumatoid arthritis, scleroderma)	Characteristic clinical picture accompanied by positive serology (see Sections 1.11, pp. 22–24, 1.13, pp. 26–28 and 1.19, pp. 39–41)
Tuberculous aortitis	Causes aneurysms rather than stenoses
	Look for evidence of TB elsewhere—chest radiograph, Mantoux test, sputum for acid-fast bacilli
Syphilitic aortitis	Very rare but worth considering
	Causes aneurysms rather than stenoses
	Check treponemal serology
Fibromuscular dysplasia	Proliferation of fibrous tissue in the media of large arteries
	Probably congenital in origin but produces progressive stenoses in young adulthood
	May be multifocal
	Non-inflammatory: unresponsive to steroids
Atherosclerosis	Rare cause of absent pulses in young people
	Consider in the presence of hyperlipidaemia

Table 18 Differential diagnosis of fever and absent radial pulses.

Clinical approach

Absent pulses on a background of fever and general ill-health in a young Asian woman immediately raises the question of vasculitic process, particularly Takayasu's arteritis. Other disorders that may cause diagnostic confusion (Table 18) should be considered and distinguished on the basis of their distinctive features. Acute arterial embolism is rendered unlikely by the length of the history. Coarctation of the aorta that is sufficiently proximal to reduce both radial pulses is rare.

History

Are there clues to suggest any of the diagnoses listed in Table 18? The most likely is Takayasu's arteritis. Assess extent and severity of arteritis by enquiring about the following:
• Systemic constitutional features suggesting active disease: fever, myalgia, lethargy, weight loss
• Specific ischaemic features: upper arm claudication, transient ischaemic (cerebral) attacks, pain over carotid arteries (carotodynia).

Examination

General

Note the temperature, weight and pallor.

Cardiovascular

Look for objective evidence of arterial occlusion:
• Listen for arterial bruits over carotids, subclavian and renal arteries
• Check for asymmetrical pulses and BP readings in both arms and legs.

 Some patients with Takayasu's arteritis may present with absent pulses and/or hypertension without constitutional symptoms.

Approach to investigations and management

Investigations

Investigations should be aimed at documenting her acute phase response as an indirect measure of disease activity, excluding other possible diagnoses, and appropriate imaging to document the extent of vascular involvement.

Serology

Both CRP and ESR are elevated in 50–70% of cases. Autoantibodies (e.g. ANA and ANCA) are not a feature of Takayasu's arteritis.

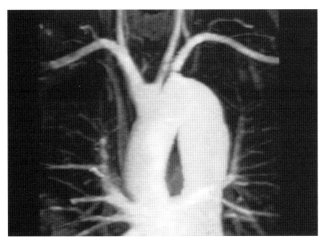

Fig. 26 MR aortic arch angiogram in a young woman with Takayasu's arteritis, depicting occlusion of the left subclavian artery at its origin. (Courtesy of Dr H Marzo-Orteza.)

Aortic arch angiography

The procedure of choice to detect arterial obstruction is angiography (Fig. 26). This is also helpful in differentiating congenital aortic coarctation from Takayasu's arteritis.

Non-invasive imaging techniques

Ultrasonography, computed tomography and MRI all provide useful information regarding aortic wall thickness. MRI is increasingly the imaging modality of choice for the serial evaluation of lesions [1].

Arterial biopsy

Such a biopsy is seldom required for the diagnosis.

 The usual biopsy finding in Takayasu's arteritis is a granulomatous panarteritis, underlining the difficulty in differentiating this condition from giant cell arteritis [2].

Management

The following are the important principles:
- Medical suppression of inflammation
- Control of hypertension
- Intervention to correct stenotic lesions (in selected cases).

Inflammation

Corticosteroids are the treatment of choice for active Takayasu's arteritis; additional immunosuppressive therapy (azathioprine, cyclophosphamide or methotrexate) is required for patients who fail to respond to steroids. Monitor response to therapy using CRP/ESR.

Hypertension

Management is with aggressive antihypertensive therapy.

Surgery

Surgery may be required in up to 50% of patients. Indications include:
- Critical renal artery stenosis causing hypertension
- Severe carotid stenosis
- Significant aortic regurgitation.

 Karam EZ, Muci-Mendoza R, Hedges TR. Retinal findings in Takayasu's arteritis. *Acta Ophthalmol Scand* 1999; 77: 209–13.
1 Flamm SD, Van Dyke C, White RD, Hoffman GS. Novel magnetic resonance imaging (MRI) techniques for evaluating active arterial inflammation in Takayasu's disease (TD). *Arthritis Rheum* 1996; 39(suppl): S201.
2 Michel BA, Arend WP, Hunder GG. Clinical differentiation between giant cell (temporal) arteritis and Takayasu's arteritis. *J Rheumatol* 1996; 23: 106–11.

2 Diseases and treatments

2.1 Immunodeficiency

2.1.1 PRIMARY ANTIBODY DEFICIENCY

Aetiology/pathophysiology/pathology

Common variable immunodeficiency (CVID) is an acquired antibody deficiency [1]. It comprises a heterogeneous group of diseases in which B cells are present (Fig. 27) but which fail to produce IgG, IgA and sometimes IgM. Some variants are associated with sarcoid-like granulomas. Autoimmunity (organ specific and haematological) is common. There may be coexistent T-cell defects.

Evidence against an intrinsic B-cell defect in CVID

- B cells in CVID are capable of secreting immunoglobulins *in vitro* with appropriate stimulation
- Infection with viruses (HIV, hepatitis C) can reverse hypogammaglobulinaemia in CVID.

Epidemiology

The incidence is estimated at 1 : 10 000–1 : 50 000. It may be sporadic or inherited in an autosomal dominant manner with variable phenotype; affected family members may have autoimmunity alone, IgA or IgG subclass deficiencies, or CVID. Ninety-five per cent present in adulthood.

Clinical presentation

Common

Complications of antibody deficiency

Complications are bacterial infections, especially of the respiratory and gastrointestinal tracts and the skin (Fig. 28).

Autoimmunity

- Organ-specific, especially thyroid disease and pernicious anaemia
- Haematological: anaemia, neutropenia, thrombocytopenia
- Arthritis: reactive or septic, particularly *Mycoplasma* sp.

B cells in CVID exhibit a curious paradox

Despite their inability to mount antibody responses to exogenous antigens, patients with CVID mount antibody responses to self-antigens, resulting in autoimmune disease.

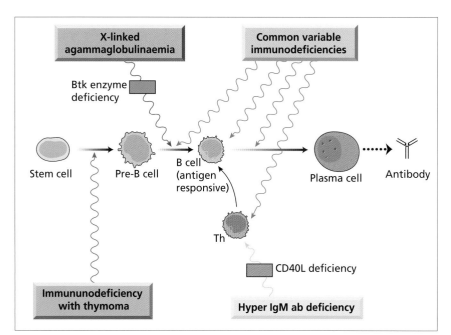

Fig. 27 Overview of the steps in B-cell maturation and the levels at which more common defects in antibody production may occur. (With permission from Chapel *et al. Essentials of Clinical Immunology*, 4th edn. Oxford: Blackwell Science, 1999.)

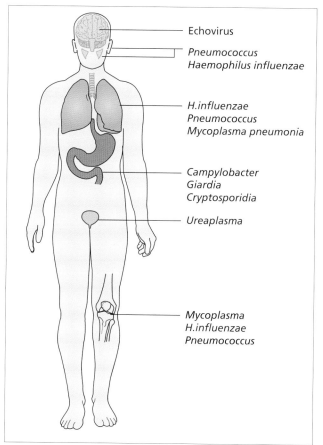

Fig. 28 Infectious complications of common variable immunodeficiency. (Courtesy of Dr ADB Webster.)

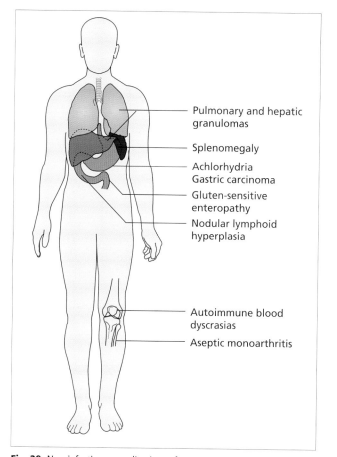

Fig. 29 Non-infectious complications of common variable immunodeficiency. (Courtesy of Dr ADB Webster.)

Granulomas

These include lung infiltrates and hepatosplenomegaly (Fig. 29).

Uncommon

• Coeliac-like enteropathy
• Diseases associated with T-cell deficiencies such as herpes zoster.

Rare

• Nodular lymphoid hyperplasia
• Thymoma.

Physical signs

Common

• Signs of bronchiectasis (see *Respiratory medicine*, Section 2.4)
• Lymphadenopathy, hepatosplenomegaly
• Arthritis
• Thyroid enlargement.

Uncommon

• Wasting.

Investigation

• Serum immunoglobulins (IgG, -A, -M). IgG subclasses are of limited value. Assess severity of antibody deficiency by measuring antibodies to past immunizations (tetanus, diphtheria) and common pathogens (*Streptococcus pneumoniae, Haemophilus influenzae* type b). If baseline antibody levels are low, proceed to test immunization and measure antibody levels in 4 weeks.
• CD3, -4, -8, -19 lymphocyte markers (to quantify total, helper and cytotoxic T-cell and B-cell numbers, respectively). Most patients with CVID have normal numbers of circulating B cells; a minority have no B cells and clinically resemble X-linked agammaglobulinaemia.
• Blood count and differential.

Differential diagnosis

• Secondary antibody deficiencies: drugs (gold, penicillamine, cytotoxics, antiepileptics); associated with lymphoproliferative disease; post-bone marrow transplantation.

- Bruton's (X-linked) agammaglobulinaemia: peak age of presentation 4 months to 2 years of age. Absent B cells, absent lymphoid tissue, no granulomas or autoimmune disease.
- Combined immunodeficiencies: T-cell-associated infections more prominent (see Section 2.1.2, pp. 56–58); usually present in childhood.

Hyper-IgM syndrome

- CD40 ligand deficiency
- X-linked
- Low IgG, high or normal IgM
- T-cell numbers normal but functionally defective with high risk of long-term opportunistic infection, particularly pneumocystis pneumonia or cryptosporidial sclerosing cholangiitis
- Bone marrow transplantation should be considered.

X-linked lymphoproliferative disease (Duncan's syndrome)

SAP (signalling lymphocyte-activating, molecule-associated protein) defect usually presenting with overwhelming Epstein–Barr virus infection or lymphoma, but occasionally with a CVID-like picture.

Treatment

Emergency

Prompt treatment of all infections, with high-dose, prolonged course (typically 2 weeks for bacterial chest infection) of antibiotics.

Long term

Regular intravenous immunoglobulin therapy at 3- to 4-weekly intervals (see Section 3.7, pp. 110–111), with or without prophylactic antibiotics. Aim to achieve trough serum IgG levels well within the normal range [2].

 Trough serum IgG levels maintained at >5 g/L prevents deterioration in lung function.

Complications

Common

- Bronchiectasis secondary to recurrent infection
- Anaemia, thrombocytopenia, neutropenia (haematological autoimmunity, splenomegaly, vitamin deficiencies resulting from malabsorption).

Uncommon

- Increased risk of lymphoma (23- to 100-fold)
- Gastric carcinoma (50-fold increase).

 Difficulties in the diagnosis of lymphoma in CVID

Lymph-node biopsies in patients with CVID may reveal bizarre histology mimicking lymphoma [3]. Biopsies should therefore be reported by a histopathologist experienced in examining tissue from patients with immune deficiency.

Rare

- Severe opportunistic infections caused by T-cell deficiency such as pneumocystis pneumonia.

Prognosis

Morbidity

- 75% suffer frequent or chronic infections
- 14% have structural damage, such as bronchiectasis.

Mortality

The mean age at death for all antibody deficiencies is 40.5 years, but the range is wide. Main causes of death are sepsis, chronic lung disease, lymphoma and other malignancies.

Prevention

Mean delay in diagnosis of 7.5 years accounts for a great deal of the morbidity and mortality. Serum immunoglobulins should be checked in anyone with unusually severe, prolonged or recurrent bacterial infections, or granulomatous disease.

1 Cunningham-Rundles C, Bodian C. Common variable immunodeficiency: clinical and immunological features of 248 patients. *Clin Immunol* 1999; 92: 34–48.
2 Chapel HM. Fortnightly review. Consensus on diagnosis and management of antibody deficiencies. *BMJ* 1994; 308: 581–585.
3 Sander CA, Medeiros LJ, Weiss LM *et al.* Lymphoproliferative lesions in patients with common variable immunodeficiency syndrome. *Am J Surg Pathol* 1992; 12: 1170–1182.

2.1.2 COMBINED T- AND B-CELL DEFECTS

Aetiology/pathophysiology/pathology

Inherited genetic defects result in failure of normal development or maturation of T lymphocytes and B

Time of presentation	Disorder	Key features
Presenting as SCID during infancy	Adenosine deaminase (ADA) deficiency*	Marked T- + B-cell lymphopenia, ↓ serum Ig Autosomal recessive
	Common cytokine receptor γ chain deficiency (γ chain shared by IL2, IL4, IL7, IL9, IL15)	Marked T-cell lymphopenia, ↓ serum Ig, normal or ↑ B-cell numbers, X-linked
	JAK 3 (Janus kinase) deficiency	As for cytokine receptor γ chain deficiency Autosomal recessive
	Recombinase activating gene (RAG$_{1/2}$) deficiency	Marked T- +B-cell lymphopenia, ↓ serum Ig
	Omenn syndrome	↑ Serum IgE, eosinophilia, ↓ serum Ig, B-cell numbers normal or ↓
	IL2 receptor α-chain deficiency	T-cell lymphopenia, serum Ig and B-cell numbers normal
	Purine nucleoside phosphorylase deficiency	T-cell lymphopenia, ↓ serum urate, serum Ig normal or ↓
Presenting in later life, including adulthood	X-linked hyper-IgM	↓ Serum IgG, IgA with ↑ or normal IgM

Table 19 Combined immunodeficiency disorders.

*Milder forms of SCID may present in adulthood, e.g. ADA deficiency.

lymphocytes, or the build up of metabolites toxic to developing lymphocytes (Table 19). Without T-cell help, production of antibody by B cells is severely limited.

Epidemiology

These defects are a heterogeneous group of conditions. They usually have autosomal recessive or sex-linked inheritance. The incidence of SCID is estimated to be 1 : 100 000 live births in France.

Clinical presentation

Common

- Presents in infancy
- Recurrent infections, sometimes with unusual 'opportunistic' organisms (see below); slow response to treatment
- Pneumonia, skin infections, eczema and persistent diarrhoea
- Failure to thrive
- Features of associated syndromes.

 Persistent lymphopenia in an ill baby is an important clue pointing towards SCID.

Uncommon

- Graft-versus-host disease (GVHD) from immuno-competent maternal cells or transfused blood. Invasive disease from BCG given at birth.

Rare

- Adult presentation: usually milder phenotype
- Papilloma viruses: warts, or cervical or anal intra-epithelial neoplasia (CIN, AIN)
- Herpes viruses: herpes simplex 1 and 2, severe varicella-zoster, Epstein–Barr virus-associated disease
- Lymphoproliferation and lymphomas
- JC virus: associated with progressive encephalopathy
- Bacterial infections, especially respiratory tract and intracellular bacteria such as *Salmonella* spp.
- Mycobacterial disease, including tuberculosis.
- Fungal infections: mucocutaneous candida infection, pneumocystis pneumonia, invasive (Fig. 30) cryptococci

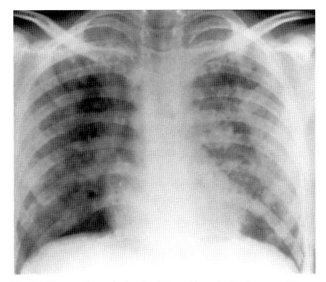

Fig. 30 Chest radiograph showing bilateral lung shadowing caused by *Pneumocystis carinii* pneumonia.

- Protozoal disease: cryptosporidial diarrhoea and cholangitis, toxoplasma cerebral abscess.

Physical signs

Common

- Poor growth and structural organ damage from repeated infections
- Active infections often present.

Investigations

See Section 3.3, pp. 102–103.

Differential diagnosis

- Secondary immunodeficiency: HIV, lymphoid malignancy.

Treatment

Short term

- Avoid live vaccines
- Irradiate blood products
- Active diagnosis and early, aggressive treatment of infections.

> To avoid GVHD, blood products should be irradiated before transfusion in patients with suspected cellular immune defects.

Long term

Prophylaxis of infection

- Intravenous immunoglobulin
- Antibiotic (co-trimoxazole) provides cover against pneumocystis and bacterial infections.

Correction of defect

- In some cases enzyme replacement (e.g. in adenosine deaminase deficiency) may be possible, but success is limited
- Consider bone marrow transplantation if HLA-match is available; success rates are, however, low in adults
- Gene therapy shows promise for the future [1].

Complications

- Vasculitis resulting from immune dysregulation
- Structural damage from recurrent infections
- Malignancy, especially lymphoma.

Prognosis

Morbidity

- Severe, from recurrent infections.

Mortality

Most affected individuals die in infancy or early childhood. For those surviving until adulthood, prognosis is poor. Death occurs from uncontrolled infection or malignancy.

Prevention

Prenatal diagnosis is often possible [2]. Fetal bone marrow transplantation is experimental and has had only limited success. Early bone marrow transplantation in selected affected infants has resulted in higher success rates [3].

Disease associations

Combined immunodeficiencies often occur in association with other congenital disease, particularly cardiac, haematological, neurological (including learning difficulties) or skeletal (including dysmorphic facies) [4].

1 Candotti F, Blaese RM. Gene therapy. In: Ochs HD, Smith CIE, Puck JM, eds. *Primary Immunodeficiency Diseases. A molecular and genetic approach.* Oxford: Oxford University Press: 1998: 476–490.
2 Jones AM, Gaspar HB. Immunogenetics: changing the face of immunodeficiency. *J Clin Pathol* 2000; 53: 60–65.
3 Buckley RH, Fischer A. Bone marrow transplantation for primary immunodeficiency diseases. In: Ochs HD, Smith CIE, Puck JM, eds. *Primary Immunodeficiency Diseases. A molecular and genetic approach.* Oxford: Oxford University Press, 1998: 459–475.
4 Ming JE, Stiehm ER, Graham JM Jr. Immunodeficiency as a component of recognizable syndromes. *Am J Med Gen* 1996; 66: 378–398.

2.1.3 CHRONIC GRANULOMATOUS DISEASE

Aetiology/pathophysiology/pathology

Inherited defect of one of four *phox* genes, which encode subunits of NADPH oxidase, the enzyme that catalyses the phagocyte respiratory burst (Fig. 31) [1], resulting in defective killing of engulfed organisms.

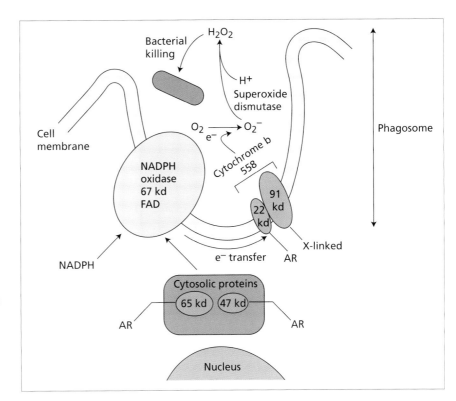

Fig. 31 Diagrammatic representation of components of the NADPH oxidase system within a phagosome, depicting bacterial killing and site of abnormalities in chronic granulomatous disease. AR, autosomal recessive; NADPH, nicotinamide adenine dinucleotide phosphate; FAD, flavin adenine dinucleotide. (Modified from *JAMA* 1990; 263: 1533–1537.)

Epidemiology

• Rare—1 : 250 000
• 67% present in infancy, but diagnosis is occasionally delayed until early adulthood
• 65% X-linked, 35% autosomal recessive inheritance.

Clinical presentation

Common

Infections

• Pneumonia, lymphadenitis, skin infections, hepatic abscesses, osteomyelitis, perianal suppuration and enteric infections
• Organisms are usually catalase positive (Table 20).

Granulomas

As chemotaxis and phagocytosis are unimpaired,

Table 20 Common pathogens in chronic granulomatous disease.

Bacteria	Fungi
Staphylococcus spp.	*Aspergillus* spp.
E. coli	*Candida* spp.
Salmonella spp.	
Klebsiella spp.	
Serratia spp.	
Burkholderia spp.	

ineffective killing by phagocytes results in the formation of granulomas; these manifest as lymphadenopathy, hepatosplenomegaly, Crohn's disease-like enteropathy with diarrhoea, dermatitis or obstructive hydronephrosis.

Miscellaneous

• Anaemia of chronic disease
• Gingivitis
• Asymptomatic chorioretinopathy [2].

Investigations

Screen with the NBT test (see Fig. 6, p. 12) or dihydrorhodamine fluorescence test (see Section 1.5, p. 12). If the screening test is abnormal, check for presence of NADPH oxidase subunits and associated gene defects.

 The NBT screening test may be misleadingly normal in some patients with CGD. Proceed to flow cytometric evaluation of the respiratory burst and genetic studies in case of diagnostic doubt.

Differential diagnosis

• Idiopathic abscesses without obvious immunodeficiency
• Crohn's disease
• Neutrophil glucose-6-dehydrogenase, myeloperoxidase or glutathione peroxidase deficiency.

Prevention

Avoid BCG in close family members until the defect has been excluded.

Disease associations

- Some individuals have increased susceptibility to *Salmonella* spp.
- Occasional association with CD4 lymphopenia.

 1 Jouanguy E, Doffinger R, Dupuis S *et al*. IL-12 and IFN-γ in host defence against mycobacteria and salmonella in mice and men. *Curr Opin Immunol* 1999; 11: 346–351.

2.1.5 TERMINAL PATHWAY COMPLEMENT DEFICIENCY

Aetiology/pathophysiology/pathology

- Inherited deletion of terminal complement (C5–9) gene
- Lack of complement-mediated lysis results in inefficient clearance of neisserial infections.

Epidemiology

- Autosomal recessive inheritance.

Clinical presentation

Common

- Recurrent invasive meningococcal disease
- Asymptomatic relative.

 Primary complement deficiency with meningococcal infection

The following are pointers towards primary complement deficiency in patients with meningococcal infection [1]:
- Unusual meningococcal serotype
- Recurrent disease
- Family history of meningococcal disease.

Uncommon

- Disseminated gonococcal disease.

Physical signs

There are usually no physical signs specifically associated with complement deficiency.

Investigations

Assess integrity of complement pathway by checking

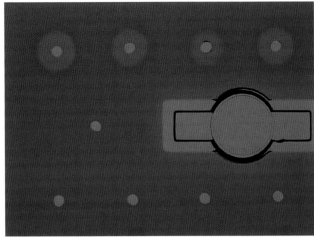

Fig. 33 Classical pathway, haemolytic complement screening test for complement deficiency. This test measures the ability of complement in the patient's serum to lyse antibody-coated erythrocytes via the classical pathway. The coated erythrocytes are embedded in a gel. Control and test sera are placed in wells and left overnight. Normal sera containing complement components C1–9 lyse the erythrocytes—seen as a ring around the well (top wells). Sera that are completely deficient in one or more complement components do not cause lysis (middle and bottom rows).

haemolytic complement activity (classical pathway CH50, alternative pathway AP50). Absence or marked reduction of both CH50 and AP50 suggests deficiency of terminal complement proteins C5–9 (Fig. 33) (see Table 1, p. 6).

 • Complement proteins are labile
• Samples for haemolytic complement activity should therefore be sent to the laboratory immediately.

Differential diagnosis

- Consider external connection to subarachnoid space: head injury, erosive sinus disease, after pituitary surgery
- Properdin [2] or factor D deficiency (check AP50)
- Other immunodeficiency.

Treatment

Emergency

This involves the prompt treatment of neisserial infection (see *Infectious diseases*, Sections 1.1, 1.14 and 2.5.2).

Short term

- Chemoprophylaxis of household contacts (see *Infectious diseases*, Section 1.38).

Long term

- Prophylactic antibiotics
- Meningococcal immunization.

Complications

The complications are those of neisserial disease (see *Infectious diseases*, Sections 1.1 and 1.14).

Prognosis

Meningococcal disease may not be as severe in the presence of complement deficiency. However, there is a significant risk of permanent disability or death.

Meningococcal disease tends to be less severe in complement-deficient patients, presumably reflecting the requirement for an intact complement pathway to cause bacterial endotoxin release.

Prevention

Primary

Primary prevention is by genetic counselling and screening of relatives at risk.

Other complement deficiencies
• C1q, C2 or C4 deficiency: C1q deficiency is strongly associated with SLE, followed in turn by homozygous C4 and C2 deficiency [3]. *May be ANA negative; more likely to be Ro positive.*
• Mannan-binding ligand deficiency: predisposition to bacterial infections *Usually evident only if another immunodeficiency is present.*
• C3 deficiency: predisposition to bacterial infections; glomerulonephritis.

1 Fijen CAP, Kuijper EJ, de Bulte MT *et al.* Assessment of complement deficiency in patients with meningococcal disease in the Netherlands. *Clin Infect Dis* 1999; 28: 98–105.
2 Linton SM, Morgan BP. Properdin deficiency and meningogoccal disease—identifying those most at risk. *Clin Exp Immunol* 1999; 118: 189–191.
3 Pickering MC, Walport MJ. Links between complement abnormalities and systemic lupus erythematosus. *Rheumatology* 2000; 39: 133–141.

2.1.6 HYPOSPLENISM

Aetiology/pathophysiology/pathology

The spleen is the major lymphoid organ for blood-borne antigens. Splenic macrophages remove bacteria, immune complexes and abnormal erythrocytes from the circulation [1].

Immunological consequences of asplenia
• Removal of a large reservoir of polysaccharide-responsive B cells
• Impaired clearance of encapsulated bacteria, intracellular protozoans (*Plasmodium*, *Babesia* spp.)
• Necessity for higher antibody levels for macrophages to clear encapsulated bacteria.

Clinical presentation

Common

• Asymptomatic: known because of underlying condition
• Fulminant septicaemia.

Uncommon

• Howell–Jolly bodies noted on blood film.

Rare

• Congenital asplenia, with cardiac abnormalities and biliary atresia.

Physical signs

There are usually no physical signs except for a splenectomy scar.

Investigations

• Blood film shows Howell–Jolly bodies (see Fig. 4, p. 10)—suggests functional hyposplenism. The absence of H–J bodies does not reliably exclude hyposplenism. Proceed to functional studies of splenic function (pitted red cell count, radioisotope uptake) in cases of diagnostic uncertainty
• Ultrasonography to confirm anatomical absence
• Pneumococcal, haemophilus b and meningococcal antibodies—higher antibody levels are required for protection in asplenic individuals.

Treatment

Emergency

• Urgent investigation and immediate empirical treatment of any febrile illness.

Long term

• Pneumococcal and haemophilus immunization
• Life-long penicillin prophylaxis.

Complications

Common

- Fulminant septicaemia, especially with encapsulated organisms (pneumococci, *Haemophilus influenzae* type b, meningococci).

Uncommon

- Severe malaria.

Rare

- Babesiosis
- Infection with *Capnocytophaga canimorsus* (from dog bite).

Prognosis

Mortality

There is a significant life-long risk of death from overwhelming infection.

Disease associations

- Haemoglobinopathies
- Coeliac disease
- Inflammatory bowel disease
- Bone marrow transplantation.

 1 Lortan JE. Management of asplenic patients (clinical annotation). *Br J Haematol* 1993; 84: 566–569.

2.2 Allergy

2.2.1 ANAPHYLAXIS

Aetiology/pathophysiology/pathology

The mechanisms of allergy (Fig. 34) involve the following:
- Sensitization (exposure to allergen and specific IgE production); followed by

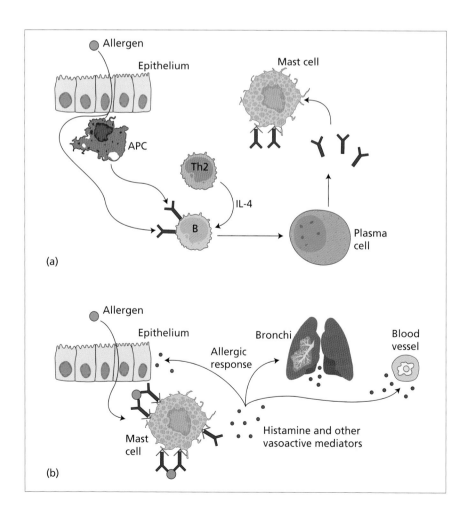

Fig. 34 Mechanism of allergy: (a) sensitization—exposure to allergen results in activation of B cell, which becomes an IgE-secreting plasma cell. Secreted IgE binds to IgE receptors on mast cells. (b) Re-exposure to the same allergen results in crosslinking of preformed allergen-specific IgE on the mast cell surface. This causes the mast cell to degranulate. The release of histamine and other vasoactive substances from the granules causes the clinical manifestations of allergy or, if severe, anaphylaxis.

• Mast cell degranulation (re-exposure to allergen binds preformed IgE on mast cell surface, inducing release of histamines and other vasoactive mediators).

Epidemiology

There are very few data on overall incidence of anaphylaxis —currently estimated at 1 : 10 000 of the population each year [1].

Common allergens include foods, drugs, insect venoms or latex.

Clinical presentation

Definition of anaphylaxis

One or more of these symptoms:
• Laryngeal oedema
• Bronchoconstriction
• Hypotension.
Anaphylaxis is caused by IgE-mediated mast cell degranulation. Abdominal cramps with severe vomiting and diarrhoea may occur. Anaphylactoid reactions are caused by non-IgE-mediated mast cell degranulation but are otherwise identical.

Common

• Facial, tongue or throat swelling
• Wheeze
• Syncope
• Feeling of impending doom.

Uncommon

• Abdominal cramps
• Diarrhoea and vomiting.

Physical signs

Common

• Urticaria, angio-oedema, skin erythema or extreme pallor
• Stridor or wheeze
• Hypotension.

Investigations

• Mast cell tryptase (within 6 h)
• Skinprick testing of suspect allergens, with positive and negative controls (Figs 35 and 36)
• IgE: total and specific to suspect allergens (RAST— radioallergosorbent test).

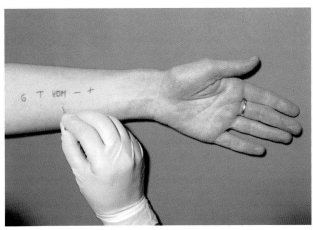

Fig. 35 Skinprick testing: a drop of a standardized extract of the suspect allergen is put on the skin. The superficial layer of the skin is lifted with a needle tip (or pricked with a lancet) through the drop. Positive (histamine) and negative (diluent) controls are included.

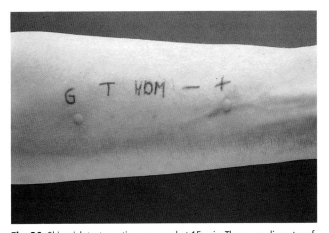

Fig. 36 Skinprick test reactions are read at 15 min. The mean diameter of the weal (not the flare) is recorded. Reactions more than 3 mm greater than the negative control are significant.

Tryptase

Tryptase levels are a marker of mast cell degranulation:
• Elevated serum β-tryptase levels are useful in differentiating anaphylactic/anaphylactoid reactions from other disorders with similar clinical manifestations [2]
• As β-tryptase is stable, stored serum or serum obtained *post mortem* should be assayed if anaphylaxis is suspected.

Differential diagnosis

• Panic attack
• Asthma
• Syncope
• C1 inhibitor deficiency
• Mastocytosis
• Ruptured hydatid cyst.

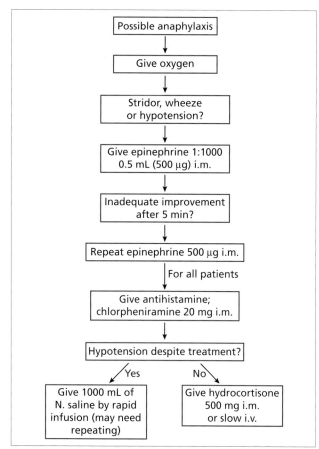

Fig. 37 Algorithm for the treatment of anaphylaxis. (Adapted from Consensus Guidelines of the Project Team of the Resuscitation Council, UK.)

Treatment

See Fig. 37.

Emergency

- Oxygen
- Intramuscular epinephrine
- Intravenous crystalloid.

Epinephrine is the drug of choice because it immediately counteracts the vasodilatation and bronchoconstriction of anaphylaxis.

Anaphylaxis in individuals on pre-existing β blockers may prove to be refractory to epinephrine. Consider use of cardiac inotropes in such cases.

Short term

- Antihistamines
- Corticosteroids.

Long term

- Identification and avoidance of allergen
- Desensitization: bee or wasp venoms and, rarely, drugs
- Patients should have a Medic-Alert bracelet and carry epinephrine in an easily injectable form (e.g. EpiPen, Ana-Kit) (see Fig. 7, p. 16).

Prognosis

Mortality

Significant numbers of deaths occur. Previously healthy young adults are often the victims.

Disease associations

- Atopy (predisposition to asthma, eczema or hayfever).

Occupational aspects

- Beekeepers (stings)
- Medical personnel (latex).

1 Stewart AG, Ewan PW. The incidence, aetiology and management of anaphylaxis presenting to an accident and emergency department. *Q J Med* 1996; 89: 859–864.
2 Joint Task Force on Practice Parameters, American Academy of Allergy, Asthma and Immunology. Evaluation and management of patients with a history of anaphylaxis. *J Allergy Clin Immunol* 1998; 101: S482–S485.

2.2.2 MASTOCYTOSIS

Aetiology

Mastocytosis encompasses a spectrum of disorders characterized by mast cell proliferation. This may be confined to the skin as in cutaneous mastocytosis or affect other organs (e.g. bone marrow, gut, bones) as in systemic mastocytosis.

The cause of mastocytosis is unknown. Normal mast cell development is dependent on interactions between the mast cell c-kit receptor (CD117) and its ligand, mast cell growth factor. Abnormalities of the c-kit receptor and its ligand are a plausible but unproven mechanism for mast cell proliferation.

Epidemiology

The precise prevalence is unknown. The estimated frequency of cutaneous mastocytosis is said to be 1 : 1000–8000 of dermatology outpatient visits.

Clinical presentation

This presentation depends on which organs are affected. Cutaneous mastocytosis is characterized by urticaria, the fixed reddish-brown maculopapules of urticaria pigmentosa (see Section 1.8, p. 17) and dermographism. Systemic mastocytosis presents with episodic flushing, diarrhoea and palpitations caused by the release of mast cell mediators. Organ infiltration may result in hepatosplenomegaly, lymphadenopathy and bone pain.

Physical signs

- Mainly confined to urticaria and the pigmented plaques of urticaria pigmentosa
- Dermographism and Darier's sign may be present.

Investigation

The key investigations are to demonstrate mast cell proliferation on skin and bone marrow trephine biopsies, coupled with biochemical evidence of elevated mast cell mediators—plasma tryptase and urinary methylhistamine.

Establish the presence of mast cells in systemic mastocytosis
- Immunophenotyping using monoclonal antibodies to CD117 and mast cell tryptase is useful in distinguishing atypical mast cells from basophils.

Differential diagnosis

See Table 6, p. 17.

Treatment

See Section 1.8, pp. 17–18.

Prognosis

In general, systemic mastocytosis progresses very slowly. For the small minority who develop an associated myelo- or lymphoproliferative disorder, the prognosis depends on the haematological disorder.

Bain BJ. Systemic mastocytosis and other mast cell neoplasms (review). *Br J Haematol* 1999; 106: 9–17.

2.2.3 NUT ALLERGY

Aetiology/pathophysiology/pathology

Nut allergy is due to IgE-mediated mast cell degranulation precipitated by contact with peanuts (strictly speaking these are pulses not nuts) or tree nuts (brazil, almond, walnut or hazelnut) (see Fig. 34).

Epidemiology

Nut allergy is more common in atopic individuals. It follows sensitization to nut(s), usually in early childhood.

Clinical presentation

Common

- Lip tingling, swelling, angio-oedema, urticaria
- Anaphylaxis, with laryngeal oedema or bronchoconstriction.

Rare

- Anaphylaxis with hypotension.

Investigations

- Detailed dietary history
- Skinprick testing or specific serum IgE measurements
- Oral challenge if diagnosis remains uncertain.

 Skinprick and challenge testing should take place where there are facilities for resuscitation, ideally in an allergy clinic.

Differential diagnosis

- Allergy to other foods
- C1 inhibitor deficiency.

Treatment

Emergency

If anaphylaxis occurs, the emergency treatment is as follows:
- Intramuscular epinephrine (see Section 2.2.1, p. 66)
- Antihistamines
- Corticosteroids.

Long term

- Avoidance of allergen.

Prognosis

Mortality

This is unknown, but there are several deaths each year in the UK.

Type	Mechanism	Clinical picture	Examples
I	Immediate hypersensitivity	Anaphylaxis Urticaria and angio-oedema Bronchospasm	Penicillins
II	Cytotoxic antibodies	Haematological cytopenias	Penicillins Heparin
III	Immune complex	Drug-induced lupus Vasculitis Serum sickness	Minocycline Carbimazole
IV	T-cell mediated	Contact dermatitis Interstitial nephritis	Topical antibiotics NSAIDs Halothane Hepatitis

Table 21 Immunological classification of drug hypersensitivity.

NSAIDs, non-steroidal anti-inflammatory drugs.

Prevention

Primary

Avoidance of contact with nuts in infancy and childhood, especially if there is a family history of atopy. Peanut products may be hidden in processed foods or creams and ointments (such as arachis oil).

Secondary

- Avoidance—detailed dietary advice is required
- Self-injectable epinephrine (see Fig. 7, p. 16) [1].

Disease associations

- Asthma
- Hayfever
- Eczema.

 Patients with food allergy and poorly controlled asthma are at particular risk of anaphylaxis.

Further allergies

Other allergies [2] may include the following:
- Tree nuts (common even if main allergy is to peanuts)
- Other foods (egg, milk, fresh fruit)
- Common air-borne allergens (pollen, house dust mite, animal dander, moulds)
- Pulses (peas, lentils, beans).

 1 Sampson H. Managing peanut allergy (Editorial). *BMJ* 1996; 312: 1050–1051.
2 Ewan P. A clinical study of peanut and nut allergy: new features and associations. *BMJ* 1996; 312: 1074–1078.

2.2.4 DRUG ALLERGY

Aetiology/pathophysiology/pathology

Immunological reactions to drugs can be classified according to the four subtypes of hypersensitivity [1] (Table 21) (see *Immunology and immunosuppression*, Sections 3–7). However, the immunological mechanisms underlying many drug reactions, particularly those affecting the skin, remain unclear. In practice, the line between immunological and non-immunological reactions to drugs is often blurred. Non-immunological adverse reactions to drugs are discussed in *Clinical pharmacology*, Section 4.

Susceptibility to drug reactions is poorly understood, but genetic factors have been identified for some drug-induced syndromes, e.g. genetically determined slow acetylation of the triggering drug is associated with drug-induced lupus and with co-trimoxazole sensitivity in HIV. Some immunological diseases are also associated with an increased risk of adverse drug reactions, particularly HIV infection and SLE.

Epidemiology

Incidence figures vary enormously from drug to drug. Crude estimates suggest that between 1% and 10% of prescriptions are complicated by some form of allergic adverse reaction.

Clinical presentation

Drug hypersensitivity can affect any system of the body and mimic many other forms of disease (Table 22). Cutaneous drug reactions are discussed in *Dermatology*, Section 2.6.

Investigations

The diagnosis of drug allergy is based largely on the history and the recognition of typical patterns of drug

Table 22 Drug reactions that mimic other syndromes.

Syndrome	Examples of triggering drugs
Systemic lupus	Minocycline
	Hydralazine
Myasthenia gravis	D-Penicillamine
Pemphigus	D-Penicillamine
Pulmonary fibrosis	Amiodarone
	Nitrofurantoin
	Some cytotoxics
Pulmonary eosinophilia	NSAIDs
	Antibiotics
Vasculitis	Antibiotics
	Thiazides
	Carbimazole
Immune haemolytic anaemia	Methyldopa
	Penicillin
Neutropenia	Carbimazole
Thrombocytopenia	Gold salts
	Diuretics
	Heparin

NSAIDs, non-steroidal anti-inflammatory drugs.

reaction, e.g. acute interstitial nephritis and toxic erythema of the skin are highly suggestive of drug reactions.

When there is a mild reaction to a therapeutically important drug, drug challenge is sometimes justified, but this must always be used cautiously. Skin tests (a local form of challenge testing) can be useful in immediate hypersensitivity (anaphylaxis) and contact dermatitis induced by topical medication.

Skin testing

Skin testing in suspected drug allergy is useful for the following agents [2]:
- Antibiotics: penicillins, cephalosporins
- Anaesthetic drugs: neuromuscular blocking agents (muscle relaxants), thiopental (thiopentone)
- Enzymes: streptokinase, chymopapain
- Chemotherapeutic agents: cisplatin
- Others: insulin, latex.

Note that false-positive and false-negative reactions may occur.

Detection of drug-specific IgE has been described in some types of drug-induced anaphylaxis, particularly to the penicillins, but is unreliable. No other clinically useful blood tests for drug allergy have been described.

Allergic to penicillin

A negative skin test to both the major and minor determinants of penicillin suggests that a patient is unlikely to develop anaphylaxis on exposure [3].

Differential diagnosis

Beware of drug reactions that mimic idiopathic systemic diseases, e.g. SLE (see Table 22).

Treatment

- Supportive care depending on organ system involved
- Treatment of immediate hypersensitivity: antihistamine and epinephrine
- Other forms of hypersensitivity: consider corticosteroids
- The overwhelming majority of reactions will resolve on drug withdrawal.

1 Borish L, Tilles SA. Immune mechanisms of drug allergy. *Immunol Allergy Clin North Am* 1998; 18: 717–729.
2 Vervloet D, Durham S. ABC of allergies: adverse reactions to drugs. *BMJ* 1998; 316: 1511–1514.
3 Sogn DD, Evans R, Shepherd G *et al.* Results of the National Institute of Allergy and Infectious Diseases Collaborative Clinical Trial to test the predictive value of skin testing with major and minor penicillin derivatives in hospitalized adults. *Ann Intern Med* 1992; 152: 1025–1032.

2.3 Rheumatology

2.3.1 CARPAL TUNNEL SYNDROME

This is the most common entrapment neuropathy; it presents commonly in rheumatology clinics.

Aetiology/pathophysiology/pathology

The median nerve is easily compromised in the tight space of the carpal tunnel. Anything that makes the space tighter will induce the carpal tunnel syndrome. The following are important causes.

Tendon swelling

- Overuse/trauma
- Rheumatoid disease.

Increased extracellular matrix or fluid retention

- Pregnancy
- Other hormonal changes: oral contraceptives
- Diabetes mellitus
- Myxoedema

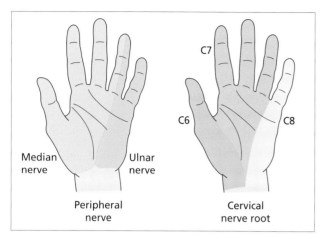

Fig. 38 Sensory innervation of the palmar surface of the hand.

- Acromegaly
- Amyloid.

Wrist arthritis

- Osteoarthritis
- Rheumatoid disease.

In many cases, particularly in women, no underlying cause will be identified. A mononeuritis in systemic vasculitis may also sometimes produce a median nerve lesion. Leprosy is a rare but important cause.

Clinical presentation

The median nerve receives sensory input from the lateral aspect of the palm (Fig. 38). However, symptoms are often more diffuse than this. The patient often describes paraesthesia in the whole hand or even extending up the arm, which is usually uncomfortable and often painful (pain may also be the result of the underlying cause). The symptoms are usually worse at night and early in the morning, and a history of nocturnal paraesthesia alone should suggest the carpal tunnel syndrome. Motor symptoms are usually less prominent, although the hand may feel generally weak.

Physical signs

It should be emphasized that examination may be entirely normal if the symptoms are intermittent (usually nocturnal). Fixed sensory changes, weakness of thumb abduction and wasting of the thenar eminence are usually only found in severe cases, and in the case of wasting, long-standing, median nerve compression.

Two provocation tests are often used:
- Percussion over the median nerve: Tinel's test
- Maintenance of fixed flexion of the wrist: Phalen's test.

These tests are positive if they produce transient sensory disturbance with a similar quality to the original symptoms. If positive, they are of good predictive value.

Investigations

A definitive diagnosis can be made using nerve conduction studies, although these may sometimes be normal in very mild intermittent compression. Electrophysiology is not obligatory in every case. Use only where the diagnosis is uncertain, or where the result will affect your management. Many surgeons require electrophysiological confirmation before carpal tunnel decompression.

- Consider also investigation of underlying cause—have a very low threshold for thyroid function testing
- Occasionally histology of the contents of the carpal tunnel will be useful, e.g. in amyloidosis.

Differential diagnosis

Cervical root compression (C5–6) and peripheral neuropathy are the main differential diagnoses. Ulnar nerve lesions are easy to distinguish by the pattern of sensory disturbance.

Treatment

This is dictated by the severity of symptoms. Many mild cases with occasional symptoms need no treatment. Conversely, intervention will be needed in most cases with severe unremitting symptoms. Most cases lie somewhere in between:
- Night-time splintage of the wrists is often used in mild compression, although there is little evidence that this is effective.
- Surgical decompression is the definitive treatment and is highly effective unless permanent nerve damage has occurred, usually in severe, long-standing cases (possibly predictable from electrophysiology).
- Injection of corticosteroids into the carpal tunnel is a simple outpatient treatment that may produce prolonged relief of symptoms, particularly in cases of recent onset or with an underlying inflammatory cause.

1 Fam AG. Common clinical problems: the upper limb in adults. In: *Oxford Textbook of Rheumatology* (Maddison PJ, Isenberg DA, Woo P, Glass DN, eds). Oxford: Oxford University Press, 1998: 135–149.
2 Hazelman B. Soft tissue rheumatism. In: *Oxford Textbook of Rheumatology* (Maddison PJ, Isenberg DA, Woo P, Glass DN, eds). Oxford: Oxford University Press, 1998: 1489–1514.

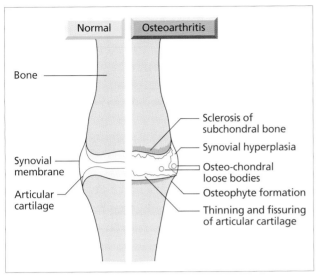

Fig. 39 Joint changes in osteoarthritis.

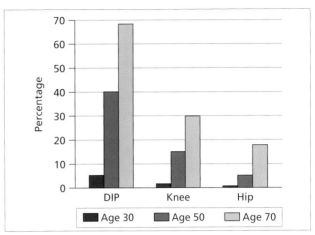

Fig. 40 Percentage prevalence of radiological changes of osteoarthritis at three different sites and at three different ages in white people living in western Europe. DIP, distal interphalangeal joint.

2.3.2 OSTEOARTHRITIS

Aetiology/pathophysiology/pathology

 Osteoarthritis is a process of joint failure rather than a disease. It can occur as a primary disorder or secondary to other insults to the joint.

The usual description of 'wear and tear' is misleading [1]. Osteoarthritis is best considered as the result of an inadequate attempt by cartilage and periarticular bone to repair itself after injury. The following are the cardinal pathological features (Fig. 39):
• Progressive disruption and loss of articular cartilage
• Remodelling of periarticular bone—usually leading to new bone formation (osteophytes in hypertrophic osteoarthritis), but sometimes to bone destruction (atrophic or erosive osteoarthritis [OA])
• Secondary changes in synovial membrane and other soft tissues
• Genetic factors are important: there is usually a strong family history in generalized nodal osteoarthritis (GNOA). The underlying genetic defects are not yet identified. OA associated with calcium pyrophosphate crystal deposition is a common feature of hereditary haemochromatosis.

Other aetiological factors include the following:
• Obesity
• Trauma or other disruptions to joint anatomy (previous fracture, congenital hip dysplasia)
• Acquired hip disease (e.g. Perthe's, slipped femoral epiphysis)
• Occupation
• Inflammatory joint disease.

Epidemiology

Osteoarthritis is very common. It can be detected radiologically in 25% of 45 year olds and virtually everyone over the age of 65 (Fig. 40). Severe disease and hand involvement are more common in women.

Clinical presentation

Osteoarthritis usually presents with pain and functional impairment, but it may be asymptomatic, particularly in the cervical and lumbar spine. Clinical features depend on the joint involved. The most common pattern of polyarticular osteoarthritis is GNOA, which is characterized by the following:
• Distal and proximal interphalangeal joint involvement
• Involvement of the base of the thumb (first carpometacarpal joint)
• Hip, knee, cervical and lumbar spine involvement
• Perimenopausal onset.

Physical signs

Tenderness, bony swelling (reflecting osteophyte formation), painful restriction of movement and crepitus are the usual findings. Note the formation of Heberden's and Bouchard's nodes in the distal and proximal interphalangeal joints, respectively. The base of the thumb often has a square appearance (see Fig. 22, p. 46). Note also the muscle wasting around affected joints and the evidence of nerve or nerve root entrapment (most commonly carpal tunnel syndrome and cervical or lumbar root entrapment—more rarely, but more seriously, spinal cord compression).

Investigations/differential diagnosis

See Section 1.22, pp. 45–47.

Treatment/prognosis

Definitive, curative medical treatment for OA remains a remote prospect. The overall outcome depends as much on muscle strength and overall fitness as on joint damage.

Osteoarthritis of the hand

Outcome in OA of the hand is usually good, with long-term function usually preserved despite pain. Pain is often worse at onset, as osteophytes grow, and tends to settle with time. Severe changes at the base of the thumb may be associated with a worse functional outcome. Surgery may be helpful in relieving pain, but is less useful in improving hand function.

Osteoarthritis of the hip and knee

Hip and knee OA is progressive only in a minority, but it may cause severe pain and disability in this subgroup. Severely impaired mobility and rest pain are the main indications for joint replacement. The outcomes from hip and knee replacement are excellent. Arthroplasty of other joints is less widely used, but the outcomes from shoulder and elbow replacement are improving.

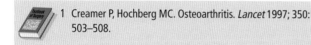

1 Creamer P, Hochberg MC. Osteoarthritis. *Lancet* 1997; 350: 503–508.

2.3.3 RHEUMATOID ARTHRITIS

Aetiology

The aetiology is unknown—current evidence supports a combination of genetic and environmental factors acting in concert [1]. There is considerable evidence for a genetic component: the risk of monozygotic twins developing rheumatoid arthritis (RA) is 12- to 62-fold higher than in unrelated individuals. There is a strong association with particular epitopes on the human leucocyte antigens HLA-DR4 and HLA-DR1 ('rheumatoid epitope' or 'shared epitope'). Over 70% of patients with erosive, seropositive disease are likely to be HLA-DR4 positive (compared with 25% of the normal population).

Epidemiology

The annual incidence in the UK is estimated to be 36 : 100 000 women and 14 : 100 000 men. Rheumatoid arthritis occurs worldwide in all ethnic groups. The peak incidence of onset is in the fifth decade.

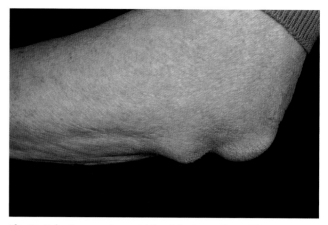

Fig. 41 Subcutaneous rheumatoid nodules in a patient with seropositive RA.

Pathology

Changes in early disease are confined to the synovial microvasculature with endothelial swelling, polymorph infiltration and thrombotic occlusion. In late disease, the synovium is heavily infiltrated by lymphocytes, macrophages and plasma cells, and it resembles an immunologically active lymph node. Rheumatoid nodules (Fig. 41) have a characteristic histological appearance with central fibrinoid necrosis surrounded by fibroblasts. Several lines of evidence suggest that T cells and macrophages play a key role in RA.

 Role of T cells and macrophages

Evidence supporting a key role for T cells and macrophages in RA:
- Synovial lymphoid infiltrates consist mainly of clonally expanded CD4+ T cells, which express markers of immunological memory (CD45 RO) and activation (CD69)
- CD4+ T cells are in close proximity to antigen-presenting cells in the synovium
- T-cell- and macrophage-derived cytokines such as IL6, TNFα and IL1 are abundantly expressed in rheumatoid joints
- Treatment with anti-TNF is of proven benefit in RA.

Clinical presentation

Common

The pattern of joint involvement is typically symmetrical, affecting hands (Fig. 42), wrists, elbows and shoulders, but usually sparing the distal interphalangeal joints. Several distinct patterns of onset are recognized (see Section 1.19, p. 39).

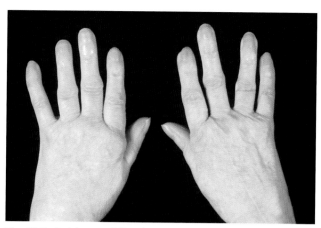

Fig. 42 Typical rheumatoid hands.

Table 23 Non-articular manifestations of rheumatoid arthritis.

System	Clinical feature
Eye	Episcleritis, scleritis, keratoconjunctivitis sicca, scleromalacia perforans (Fig. 43)
Skin	Rheumatoid nodules, vasculitis (palpable purpura), palmar erythema and pyoderma ganagrenosum
Haematological	Anaemia, splenomegaly, Felty's syndrome, lymphadenopathy and cryoglobulinaemia
Respiratory	Pleurisy with effusion, pulmonary fibrosis, Caplan's syndrome
Cardiovascular	Raynaud's phenomenon, pericarditis, myocarditis, cardiac nodules, mitral valve disease
Neurological	Carpal tunnel syndrome, peripheral neuropathy, mononeuritis multiplex, cervical myelopathy

Criteria for rheumatoid arthritis

The following are the revised criteria of the American Rheumatism Association for the classification of RA (1987):
- Morning stiffness (duration >1 h lasting >6 weeks)
- Arthritis of at least three areas (soft tissue swelling or fluid >6 weeks)
- Arthritis of hand joints (wrist, MCP joints or PIP joints >6 weeks)
- Symmetrical arthritis (at least one area >6 weeks)
- Rheumatoid nodules (as observed by physician)
- Serum rheumatoid factor
- Radiological changes (as seen on anteroposterior films of wrists and hands).

The presence of four criteria is required for diagnosis of RA.

Physical signs

Common

These are confined to acute synovitis in early RA. Joint deformities (see Fig. 17) are characteristic of chronic disease.

Uncommon

- Rheumatoid nodules
- Extra-articular manifestations (Table 23).

Investigations

The diagnosis of RA is based on a collection of clinical features, rather than on a specific pathognomonic abnormality. Investigations are helpful in assessing disease severity and prognosis.

Blood count

Red cell count

Many patients with active disease are anaemic. Aetiology of anaemia is multifactorial.

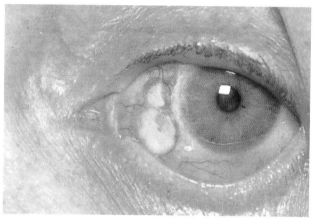

Fig. 43 Scleromalacia perforans in a patient with seropositive RA. (With permission from *Arthritis and Rheumatism in Practice*, Merck, Gower Medical Publishing.)

Causes of anaemia in RA

- Normochromic/normocytic anaemia caused by chronic disease itself
- Hypochromic/microcytic anaemia secondary to iron deficiency (↑ gastrointestinal bleeding caused by NSAIDs)
- Macrocytic anaemia resulting from folate deficiency (sulphasalazine, methotrexate) or vitamin B_{12} deficiency (associated pernicious anaemia)
- Haemolysis (drug induced by sulphasalazine and dapsone)
- Bone marrow suppression (drug induced by sulphasalazine, gold and cytotoxic agents)
- Hypersplenism as in Felty's syndrome.

White cell count

This may be normal. It is elevated in patients with severe disease, infection or on steroid therapy. Leucopenia may be drug induced or secondary to peripheral consumption, as in Felty's syndrome.

Platelet count

This is usually normal; thrombocytosis is a feature of active disease whereas thrombocytopenia may be caused by drug-induced marrow suppression or Felty's syndrome.

Acute phase indices

Both the ESR and CRP are elevated in active disease and correlate with disease severity.

Rheumatoid factor

This factor is positive in 70% of patients. High titres are usually associated with severe RA, particularly with extra-articular features.

Radiology

Small joints of the hands and feet are affected early in the disease. Typical changes include the following:
- Soft tissue swelling
- Periarticular osteoporosis
- Loss of joint space
- Marginal erosions regarded as a characteristic feature of RA.

Synovial fluid analysis

See Sections 1.19, p. 41 and 3.5, pp. 107–108.

Synovial biopsy

Synovial histology is rarely necessary and is not pathognomonic. It is sometimes useful in excluding tuberculosis in a patient with monoarticular disease.

Differential diagnosis

See Section 1.19, p. 40.

Treatment

The following are the aims of treatment:
- Relief of symptoms
- Suppression of active disease and arrest of disease progression
- Restoration of function to affected joints.

To achieve these aims, a multidisciplinary team approach is vital, encompassing rheumatologists, occupational therapists, physiotherapists, nurses, social workers and orthopaedic surgeons. Patient education is equally crucial. Ensure that the patient understands the chronicity of disease with its exacerbations and remissions.

Active phase treatment

Local measures

- Splints to rest joints
- Physiotherapy
- Intra-articular steroids (see Section 3.6, pp. 108–110). These are very useful where one or more joints continues to be painful despite simple analgesics and NSAIDs. The duration of symptomatic relief is variable (2–4 weeks).

Drug treatment

The traditional pyramidal approach to drug therapy—in which NSAIDs are used as first-line agents with late introduction of disease-modifying antirheumatic drugs (DMARDs)—is no longer valid because the assumptions (see key point below) underpinning this approach have been shown to be incorrect [2].

 The following traditional assumptions regarding drug treatment of RA are now known to be erroneous:
- RA is a benign disease
- Aspirin and NSAIDs are non-toxic therapies
- DMARDs are too toxic for routine use.

Current consensus favours the early use of DMARDs (see below) in view of:
- Their efficacy as a group in arresting disease progression
- The recognition that the risks associated with untreated disease may be greater than the toxicity of drug treatment.

NON-STEROIDAL ANTI-INFLAMMATORY DRUGS

These drugs provide symptomatic relief by suppressing inflammation, but they do not influence the underlying disease process. Most patients with RA require daily treatment. Additional simple analgesics, such as paracetamol with or without opiates, are useful if pain relief is inadequate.

DISEASE-MODIFYING ANTIRHEUMATIC DRUGS

These drugs are a heterogeneous group of drugs comprising chloroquine, sulphasalazine, gold, methotrexate, steroids, azathioprine and cyclosphophamide.

They are increasingly used early in disease (see above). DMARDs are slow-acting drugs that inhibit cytokine-mediated inflammatory damage, thereby preventing joint destruction and preserving joint function. Regular monitoring is required to prevent toxicity (Table 24).

Table 24 Side effects of DMARDs.

Drug	Side effects
Gold	Mouth ulcers, skin rash, bone marrow suppression and nitritoid reaction (flushing)
Sulphasalazine	Nausea, vomiting, mouth ulcers, bone marrow suppression and transient azoospermia
Methotrexate	Nausea, vomiting, mouth ulcers, hepatotoxicity, bone marrow suppression, renal and pulmonary damage

Steroids

These are used via either the intra-articular or the intramuscular route. Both afford temporary relief lasting 2–4 weeks. Useful in two situations:
- Acute exacerbations of disease
- As a stop-gap measure before DMARDs start acting.

Oral steroids are rarely justified, although intravenous steroid pulses are useful as a short-term measure for severe disease exacerbations, e.g. rheumatoid vasculitis.

Cytotoxic therapy

This is rarely used, usually being reserved for resistant disease.

New agents in RA treatment

COX-2 inhibitors

Celecoxib and rofecoxib selectively inhibit cyclo-oxygenase-2 (COX-2), the COX isoform that is expressed in inflammatory lesions, in contrast to COX-1 which is constitutively expressed in most tissues. COX-2 inhibitors are useful in RA because they inhibit synovial prostaglandin (PG) production while sparing intestinal PG synthesis, which is mediated by COX-1. The main advantage of COX-2 inhibitors over conventional NSAIDs is the lower risk of gastrointestinal ulceration.

Pyrimidine synthesis inhibitors

Leflunomide is a new DMARD that is as effective as methotrexate but has a reportedly lower risk of pulmonary adverse effects.

TNF inhibitors

Two types of TNF inhibitors are beneficial in resistant RA [3]. Both infliximab (a chimaeric anti-TNF antibody) and etanercept (a soluble TNF receptor) act by potently binding TNF and consequently reducing the proinflammatory effects of this cytokine.

Surgery

Joint replacement is indicated once irreversible joint damage has occurred. The overall outcome after knee and hip replacement is favourable, with promising results being seen with elbow and shoulder replacement.

Prognosis

Severe disabling disease occurs in 10%. Major causes of death are infection, vasculitis and secondary amyloidosis.

Poor prognostic factors in RA

- Female patients
- Severe disease and/or severe disability at presentation
- Extra-articular disease
- High concentration of rheumatoid factor (RF)
- Evidence of early (first 3 years) erosions on radiological examination
- HLA-DR4.

1 Weyand CM. New insights into the pathogenesis of rheumatoid arthritis. *Rheumatology* 2000; 39 (suppl 1): 3–8.
2 Fries JF. Current treatment paradigms in rheumatoid arthritis. *Rheumatology* 2000; 39 (suppl 1): 30–35.
3 Pisetsky DS. TNF blockers in rheumatoid arthritis (editorial). *N Engl J Med* 2000; 342: 810–811.

2.3.4 SERONEGATIVE SPONDYLOARTHRITIDES

Definition of seronegative spondyloarthritis [1]

Generic term for a group of rheumatological disorders characterized by:
- spinal inflammation
- synovitis (usually affecting large joints)
- mucocutaneous inflammation.
Rheumatoid factor is absent (hence seronegative).

These disorders include the following:
- Ankylosing spondylitis (features of which may occur in all the other syndromes)
- Psoriatic arthritis
- Reiter's syndrome and reactive arthritis
- Enteropathic arthritis (associated with inflammatory bowel disease).

Considerable overlap may occur between these syndromes and, in some patients, the generic label seronegative spondyloarthropathy may be more appropriate than any of the above.

Table 25 Prevalence of HLA-B27.

Disease	Percentage prevalence
UK controls	5–10
Ankylosing spondylitis	95
Reiter's syndrome/reactive arthritis	80
Psoriatic arthritis (total)	20
Psoriatic spondylitis	50

Aetiology/pathophysiology/pathology

Genetic factors are important, with HLA-B27 being the most clearly defined association (Table 25). Infectious agents (mucosal or skin) are thought to be the most important environmental trigger. This is best defined for reactive arthritis, with infectious agents including the following:

- *Chlamydia trachomatis*
- *Salmonella* spp.
- *Shigella* spp.
- *Campylobacter jejuni*
- *Yersinia enterocolitica.*

The inflammatory process probably results from an immune response against non-viable bacterial antigens sequestered in musculoskeletal tissues, perhaps leading to a secondary autoimmune response. The cardinal pathological feature is enthesitis [2], an enthesis being the junctional tissue between the muscle/ligament/tendon and bone. Enthesitis is responsible for spinal inflammation in ankylosing spondylitis and localized problems such as plantar fasciitis and Achilles' tendonitis.

Enthesitis is also probably the first pathological change in joint inflammation in these disorders.

Epidemiology

All these disorders show a male preponderance, in contrast with most chronic immunological rheumatic diseases.

Clinical presentation

General features

Common features that may occur in all spondyloarthropathies:
- Insidious onset of spinal pain and restriction
- Localized enthesitis, e.g. plantar fasciitis, Achilles' tendonitis
- Large-joint synovitis
- Acute uveitis (painful red eye).

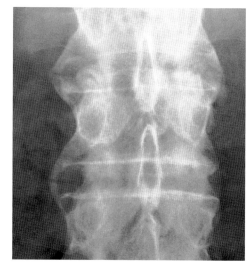

Fig. 44 Spinal fusion in ankylosing spondylitis. (Courtesy of Dr M Pattrick.)

Specific features

Ankylosing spondylitis

- Spinal symptoms predominate
- Involvement of whole spine (Fig. 44)
- May have large joint oligoarthritis in lower limbs, especially the hips.

Reactive arthritis/Reiter's syndrome

- Often begins acutely—severe systemic disturbance may be present and mimic sepsis (which should be actively excluded).
- History of diarrhoea or urethritis up to a month before the articular disease. These features are often absent, however, particularly in postchlamydial reactive arthritis. A triggering infection can be reliably identified only in about 50% of patients.
- The spectrum of disease ranges from purely articular (reactive arthritis) to multisystem (Reiter's syndrome).
- The most common presentation is acute lower limb, large joint mono- or oligoarthritis in a young male.
- Scaly psoriasis-like eruption on hands/feet—keratoderma blennorrhagica.
- Eroded appearance to glans penis—circinate balanitis.
- Conjunctivitis is more common than uveitis.

 Chlamydial genitourinary infection is often clinically silent and needs to be actively excluded in reactive arthritis.

Psoriatic arthritis

Several patterns, which may overlap (percentages are of total psoriatic arthritis population):

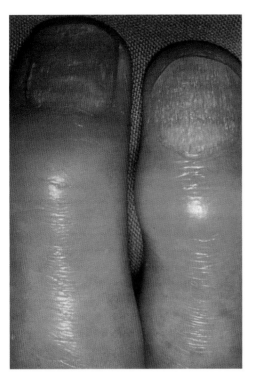

Fig. 45 Distal interphalangeal joint and nail involvement in psoriatic arthropathy. (Courtesy of Dr M Pattrick.)

- Distal interphalangeal joint (7–17%) (Fig. 45)
- Asymmetrical oligoarthritis (30–55%)
- Symmetrical polyarthritis, similar to rheumatoid arthritis (20–40%)
- Arthritis mutilans (not unlike rheumatoid, but grossly destructive, often with telescoping digits) (2–15%)
- Sacroiliitis and spondylitis (5–30%).

Dactylitis (sausage-like finger or toe swelling, usually affecting only one or two digits) is a distinctive feature, occurring in around 25% of patients. The severities of the skin and joint disease are not correlated. Some patients may have joint disease that is highly suggestive of psoriatic arthritis, but no obvious skin disease. Skin disease may appear many years later.

Enteropathic arthritis

There are two patterns (again they may overlap):
- Large-joint, lower-limb oligo- or monoarthritis—activity tends to mirror the severity of bowel inflammation
- Ankylosing spondylitis.

Uncommon features

- Aortitis, which may lead to aortic incompetence
- Pulmonary fibrosis (ankylosing spondylitis)
- Spinal discitis, which may lead to instability and spinal cord and nerve root compression
- Amyloid (as in all chronic inflammatory disease).

Physical signs

It is necessary to assess spinal disease in ankylosing spondylitis, as follows.

Lumbar spine

Restricted movement is almost always found, usually more so than in mechanical back pain, and usually in all directions. The Schober index is used for serial measurement [1].

Thoracic spine

Dorsal kyphosis often develops as disease progresses. Chest expansion is the best index: <5 cm is abnormal.

Cervical spine

This is globally restricted, with the neck being forced into a flexed position by dorsal kyphosis. When standing with his or her back to a wall, can the patient touch the wall with his or her occiput. If not, measure the occiput to wall distance.

Investigations

Synovial fluid

Microscopy and culture are essential to exclude sepsis and crystal arthritis.

Blood tests

Measures of the acute phase response are useful:
- to distinguish inflammatory from non-inflammatory back pain
- to assess disease activity/response to treatment.

Ascertainment of HLA-B27 status is of limited diagnostic value because it is present in around 5–10% of population. It may be of limited use in completing the diagnostic jigsaw.

Identifying a triggering cause

Looking for a triggering cause in Reiter's syndrome/reactive arthritis:
- *Chlamydia* spp. are the most common triggering cause, and may be clinically silent. Chlamydia serology is of little use. Diagnosis can be made only by detection of the organism in the genital tract (antigen detection or PCR). Referral to a genitourinary physician may be required.
- Diagnosis of campylobacter/shigella/salmonella infection

may be possible by culture if the patient has recent diar-rhoea, but this is unlikely to be successful if the gastrointestinal symptoms have settled

• In practice, the clinical picture is often suggestive of reactive arthritis, but no triggering organism is identified.

Think about HIV

Remember that florid Reiter's syndrome and psoriatic arthropathy may be presenting features of HIV infection.

Radiology

Sacroiliitis

This may be asymptomatic. It is worth looking for in unexplained mono- and oligoarthritis because the presence of bilateral sacroiliitis makes the diagnosis of a spondyloarthropathy very likely. Beware of unilateral sacroiliitis: this may be due to sepsis, so consider aspiration or biopsy.

Spinal radiographs

These are indicated in back pain of an inflammatory pattern. Sacroiliitis and vertebral changes may be diagnostic long before the classic bamboo spine develops.

Peripheral joint disease

Look for erosions and use to assess the progress of damage.

Occult inflammatory bowel disease

Consider small bowel radiology/large bowel endoscopy in:
• 'reactive arthritis' with persistent bowel symptoms
• erythema nodosum
• persistent mono-/oligoarthritis with an acute phase response or anaemia that seems out of proportion to the articular disease.

Differential diagnosis

• Spinal disease: beware infective or neoplastic spinal pathology, especially in the older patient. Mechanical back pain may sometimes give a very inflammatory picture.
• Monoarthritis: consider sepsis and crystal arthritis (see Section 1.18, p. 37).
• Oligoarthritis: consider crystal arthritis, rheumatic fever in the younger patient or Lyme disease if travel/

resident in endemic area. Dactylitis is also a feature of sarcoid arthropathy.
• Polyarthritis: parvovirus arthritis and other postviral arthritides, rheumatoid disease.
• Joint and mucocutaneous disease: SLE, Behçet's syndrome.
• Joint and gut disease: vasculitis, Whipple's disease, coeliac disease.

Treatment

Short term

• Exclude sepsis, symptomatic NSAIDs for pain and stiffness, intra-articular corticosteroid injections
• Treat any associated sexually transmitted infection in Reiter's syndrome/reactive arthritis (this has little or no influence on the joint disease)
• Control inflammatory bowel disease.

Long term

• Life-long daily exercise plan via physiotherapists for spinal disease
• Sulphasalazine and methotrexate useful in peripheral joint disease; little or no impact on spinal disease
• Methotrexate particularly useful in psoriatic arthritis.

Prognosis

Ankylosing spondylitis

Many patients do well, with only a minority having severely disabling disease. Joint replacement is necessary in 15% (most often hips).

Poor prognostic features in ankylosing spondylitis

• Onset in adolescence
• High acute-phase response
• Extraspinal joint disease.

Reactive arthritis/Reiter's syndrome

• Remission in more than 70% at 1 year, 85% at 2 years, but relapse can occur in 30–50%, perhaps provoked by recurrent exposure to triggering infection
• Persistent long-term disease in 10–30%
• Persistence and recurrence more likely if HLA-B27 present.

Psoriatic arthritis

The outcome of psoriatic arthritis depends on the

pattern. Asymmetrical oligoarthritis has a good long-term outcome. A mutilans picture is associated with considerable disability.

1 Calin A. Spondyloarthropathy. In: *Oxford Textbook of Rheumatology* (Maddison PJ, Isenberg DA, Woo P, Glass DN, eds). Oxford: Oxford University Press, 1998: 1037–1098 (also the following four chapters in this book).
2 McGonagle D, Khan MA, Marzo-Ortega H *et al*. Enthesitis in spondyloarthropathy. *Curr Opin Rheumatol* 1999; 11: 244–250.

2.3.5 IDIOPATHIC INFLAMMATORY MYOPATHIES

Aetiology/pathophysiology/pathology

Usual classification

- Primary idiopathic polymyositis (PM)
- Primary idiopathic dermatomyositis (DM)
- PM or DM with malignancy
- Childhood DM (not discussed here)
- PM or DM with another connective tissue disease
- Inclusion body myositis.

These myopathies are usually considered to be auto-immune disorders [1]. They are paraneoplastic in 10% of cases. The immunological mechanism of muscle damage is largely via T cells in polymyositis and antibody and complement in dermatomyositis. Striated muscle involvement predominates, although cardiac and smooth muscle can be involved. Skeletal muscle pathology usually shows lymphocytic infiltration and fibre damage.

Epidemiology

These are rare disorders, with an incidence of around $5 : 10^6$ per year. Female : male ratio is about 2 : 1, although the sexes are equally affected by paraneoplastic myositis.

Clinical presentation

Muscle

This is usually with weakness rather than pain. The assessment of the patient with proximal weakness is discussed in Section 1.15 (pp. 29–32). Non-skeletal involvement may produce cardiac failure and oropharyngeal dysfunction.

Skin

The following are three important features:

- Nail-fold capillary dilatation, usually visible to the naked eye
- The development of scaly rashes on light-exposed skin
- Angio-oedematous changes, particularly on the face.

Lung

Intercostal and diaphragmatic weakness occurs in severe cases, although respiratory failure is unusual. Interstitial lung disease, clinically indistinguishable from crytogenic fibrosing alveolitis, occurs in around a fifth of cases. The lung disease may be the presenting feature, initially with mild muscle changes.

Investigations

An assay of creatine kinase (CK) is the best marker of muscle damage, although it is not specific to myositis (see Section 1.15, p. 31). CK is a useful marker of response to treatment. PM and DM may occasionally present with a normal CK. Screening for malignancy, use of muscle biopsy, electromyography and muscle imaging are discussed under Section 1.15, pp. 31–32.

Detection of autoantibodies is often helpful, although around a third of patients with PM/DM do not have any recognized pattern of autoantibodies. The presence of high-titre ANAs greatly increases the diagnostic likelihood of PM/DM or other connective tissue diseases. A variety of distinctive patterns of autoantibody production is seen in defined subtypes of myositis and overlap syndromes [2]. These patterns are usually detected using screening tests for antibodies to extractable nuclear antigens (ENAs). These include anti-Jo-1, anti-U1RNP and anti-PM-Scl, which are all associated with syndromes that include myositis, lung disease and scleroderma-like changes.

Differential diagnosis

See Section 1.15, pp. 29–32.

Don't automatically assume that:
- A normal CK excludes myositis
- A raised CK is the result of myositis without additional investigation
- Lymphocytic infiltrates in muscle are always caused by myositis.

Treatment

Corticosteroids form the mainstay of treatment, initially at high doses. Most patients require a steroid-sparing drug (usually azathioprine) as the dose of steroids is reduced. Cyclosporin, other immunosuppressant drugs and high-dose intravenous immunoglobulin can all be used where response to treatment is poor. Assessing response to treatment is usually by serial measurement of CK and muscle strength. Physiotherapy is an important adjunct to pharmacological treatment.

> **Reassessment**
>
> Where response to treatment is poor, consider re-biopsy to reassess the following:
> • Initial diagnosis: is this really PM/DM? Inherited myopathies can sometimes be confused. Inclusion body myositis is a variant of PM that is much less responsive to immunosuppression.
> • Treatment or disease: could persistent weakness be corticosteroid induced?

Skin and lung involvement will usually respond in parallel with the muscle disease, but topical steroids and antimalarials may be useful in skin disease and more aggressive immunosuppression may be required for lung disease.

Rapid, non-specific deterioration may reflect progression of underlying malignancy rather than the muscle disease itself.

Prognosis

Morbidity

Although most will show some response to immunosuppression, the morbidity of PM and DM is high. Overall, more than 50% of patients will have some long-term muscle weakness. The response to treatment in DM and myositis associated with other connective tissue diseases is better than in PM. Onset over the age of 65 is a poor prognostic sign.

Mortality

The 5-year mortality rate is 10–15% with malignancy, infection (resulting from immunosuppression), and lung and heart disease as the major causes of death. Mortality in paraneoplastic myositis is primarily determined by the underlying malignancy.

1 Callen JP. Dermatomyositis. *Lancet* 2000; 355: 53–57.
2 Targoff IN. Polymyositis and dermatomyositis in adults. In: *Oxford Textbook of Rheumatology* (Maddison PJ, Isenberg DA, Woo P, Glass DN, eds). Oxford: Oxford University Press, 1998: 1287–1300.

2.3.6 CRYSTAL ARTHRITIS: GOUT

Aetiology/pathophysiology/pathology

> **Poorly soluble crystals**
>
> A variety of poorly soluble crystals can be found in joints [1], some of which can induce inflammation, including the following:
> • Monosodium urate—the cause of gout
> • Calcium pyrophosphate—the cause of pseudogout
> • Apatite—possibly associated with aggressive forms of osteoarthritis (rare and not discussed further here).

Formation of monosodium urate crystals is a consequence of hyperuricaemia, which in turn results from overproduction or inefficient renal excretion of uric acid, or a combination of the two. The biochemistry of uric acid formation and its relationship to cell turnover is discussed in *Biochemistry*, Section 7. Poor excretion is probably the major factor in most cases of gout. Obesity, diuretic usage and alcohol consumption are the main environmental causes, but genetic factors play a strong modulating role. Drugs are an important contributory cause, particularly diuretics and cyclosporin.

Crystals tend to form:
• in joints
• subcutaneously
• in the kidney and renal tubules.

Subcutaneous crystals tend to form discrete masses or tophi. The crystals induce inflammation by activation of leucocytes and/or the complement cascade.

Epidemiology

Gout is common, affecting more than 1% of the population, and is the most common cause of the acute hot joint. Gout is predominantly a male disease, and only occurs in significant numbers in women over the age of 60, when it is almost invariably associated with diuretic usage.

Clinical presentation

A number of overlapping syndromes are associated with urate crystal deposition:
• Acute gout
• Tophaceous gout
• Nephrolithiasis
• Uric acid nephropathy.

Acute gout

This usually presents with an episodic, self-limiting, flitting mono- or oligoarthritis, most commonly of the

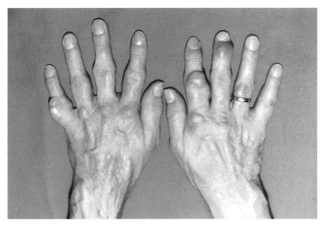

Fig. 46 Tophaceous gout in the hands of an elderly woman on diuretics.

first metatarsophalangeal joint and knee, but it can produce an asymmetrical polyarthritis. Extra-articular acute attacks can occur in bursae (especially the olecranon). The inflammation is usually severe and exquisitely painful, although polyarthritic gout tends to be less florid. The attacks may be associated with systemic ill-health and fever. Precipitants include the following:
• Alcohol excess
• Intercurrent illness (including surgery)
• Starvation
• The introduction of any drug that interferes with the handling of uric acid (including allopurinol).
   The joint generally returns to normal between attacks.

Tophaceous gout

Widespread tophus formation can occur on a background of recurrent long-standing acute gout, but it can also occur in elderly women on diuretics in the absence of acute attacks (Fig. 46). Tophi are usually pea sized, but can be very large. They tend to occur on pressure points, such as extensor surfaces, and the pinnae.

Nephrolithiasis

Uric acid crystals account for around 8% of all renal/ureteric calculi. They are radiolucent.

Uric acid nephropathy

Hyperuricaemia is a common finding in renal impairment, usually as a consequence of impaired kidney function, hypertension or drug treatment, rather than the cause. The important exception is acute uric acid nephropathy which occurs in high cell turnover states, particularly leukaemias and lymphomas in the early stages of chemotherapy. Systemic illness and poor renal perfusion increase the risk of renal failure.

Physical signs

For physical signs see Section 1.18 (pp. 36–39). Gout and sepsis are the only common causes of a red-hot joint, and it is important to differentiate the two by joint aspiration if there is any doubt. Gout may also mimic infection by producing spreading cellulitic changes, which may desquamate as recovery occurs.

Investigations

• Aspiration of synovial fluid is the only definitive diagnostic manoeuvre (see Section 1.18, p. 38). Uric acid crystals can be found in between acute attacks, and the diagnosis can be made by aspiration of a quiescent joint—only a tiny amount of fluid is required. Crystals can also be seen in material aspirated from bursae and tophi.
• Measurement of serum uric acid is of little value: hyperuricaemia is far more common than clinical gout and furthermore the level may be normal during an acute attack.
• Uric acid excretion can be used to define overproducers and underexcretors, but this is rarely of clinical value.
• Assess renal function and consider screening for common co-morbid conditions: hypertension, diabetes mellitus and hypercholesterolaemia.
• Radiographs may be useful in chronic disease: periarticular tophi produce a distinctive punched-out pattern, which can be distinguished from other erosive arthropathies.

Differential diagnosis

For more detail on this, see Section 1.18, pp. 36–39. Chronic tophaceous gout can be confused with:
• rheumatoid arthritis
• psoriatic arthritis
• nodal osteoarthritis.

Treatment

Short term

NSAIDs

NSAIDs are the mainstay of acute treatment, but beware the use of NSAIDs in renal impairment, because marked deterioration may occur.
• Indomethacin has acquired a reputation for being the most effective, but there is little evidence for this.
• Aspirin is usually avoided because it inhibits excretion of urate.

Colchicine

Colchicine is poorly tolerated and has little to recommend it as a first-line treatment.

Corticosteroids

Corticosteroids are invaluable, particularly in patients unable to tolerate NSAIDs. Intra-articular administration is preferred when one or a small number of joints are affected. Alternatively, consider a short 7- to 10-day oral burst (e.g. prednisolone 40 mg daily). Some advocate tailing off the dose over a week or two, but others do not feel that this is necessary.

Long term

Most of the predisposing causes of gout are reversible. Clearly there are good reasons for addressing these beyond the potential reduced risk of recurrent gout.

Prophylaxis

Prophylactic treatment should be considered in the following circumstances:
- Recurrent acute attacks
- Chronic tophaceous gout
- Renal impairment
- Leukaemias/lymphomas/bulky solid tumours before aggressive chemotherapy
- Inherited syndromes with uric acid overproduction, e.g. Lesch–Nyhan syndrome.

Allopurinol is the mainstay of prophylaxis, usually at a dose of 300 mg daily unless renal impairment is present. This is usually not started until around 2 weeks after an acute attack because it may initially precipitate further attacks. For this reason, a NSAID or low-dose colchicine is often co-prescribed for the first few weeks of allopurinol treatment.

Allopurinol is usually well tolerated but can provoke severe mucocutaneous reactions, including the Stevens–Johnson syndrome.

Recurrent gout on allopurinol usually reflects poor compliance or persistent high alcohol use, but some require dose increases up to 900 mg daily (aim to normalize serum urate). Uricosuric drugs (probenecid, sulphinpyrazone) are occasionally useful when allopurinol is ineffective or not tolerated.

Beware the interaction between allopurinol and azathioprine in the post-transplantation patient. Azathioprine toxicity may result because allopurinol inhibits xanthine oxidase, an enzyme responsible for metabolizing azathioprine.

1 Rosenthal AK. Crystal arthropathies. In: *Oxford Textbook of Rheumatology* (Maddison PJ, Isenberg DA, Woo P, Glass DN, eds). Oxford: Oxford University Press, 1998: 1555–1581.

2.3.7 CALCIUM PYROPHOSPHATE DEPOSITION DISEASE

Aetiology/pathophysiology/pathology

This disease is poorly understood. Pyrophosphate crystals form in articular cartilage and are shed into the synovial fluid where they can provoke an inflammatory response. Pyrophosphate crystal formation occurs increasingly with age, but is also associated with a number of metabolic disorders:
- Hereditary haemochromatosis
- Primary hyperparathyroidism
- Previous joint trauma (including surgery)
- Previous intra-articular bleeding
- Hypophosphatasia (rare inherited deficiency of alkaline phosphatase).

Epidemiology

Acute pseudogout is largely a disorder of elderly people, unless it is secondary to a metabolic disorder. Incidence is about half that of gout. Radiographic chondrocalcinosis is more common.

Clinical presentation

Acute pseudogout

This disease presents like any other acute hot joint (see Section 1.18, p. 37), often with striking fever and systemic illness. Intercurrent illness is the most common precipitant.

Chronic joint disease

The spectrum of disease ranges from a rheumatoid-like picture with synovitis to a variant of OA. There is shoulder, elbow, wrist and metacarpophalangeal joint (especially second and third) involvement in the upper limb.

Investigations

For investigations, see Section 1.18, p. 38. The rheumatoid-like picture is not associated with rheumatoid factor or usually with an acute phase response. Diagnosis of the chronic joint diseases is largely radiological—looking for chondrocalcinosis (Fig. 47) and the distinctive pattern of degenerative joint disease.

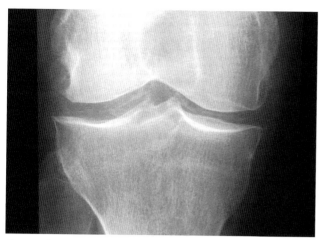

Fig. 47 Chondrocalcinosis of the knee.

 Investigate potential secondary causes, especially haemochromatosis. Ferritin, serum iron and iron binding, calcium and alkaline phosphatase should be measured in most cases, especially the younger patient.

Treatment

Acute pseudogout is best managed with NSAIDs or intra-articular steroid injection, once sepsis has been excluded. Low-dose colchicine has been used to prevent recurrent attacks. There are no specific treatments for the chronic pyrophosphate arthropathies.

2.4 Autoimmune rheumatic diseases

2.4.1 SYSTEMIC LUPUS ERYTHEMATOSUS

Aetiology/immunopathogenesis

The cause of systemic lupus erythematosus (SLE) is unknown. It has a clear genetic element as evidenced by the higher rate of concordance in monozygotic twins (25%) compared with dizygotic twins (3%). Risk factors include the HLA haplotype HLA-A1, -B8, -DR3, complement C4 null alleles and primary complement deficiency (of early components—C1q, C1r, C1s, C4, C2) [1]. Defective clearance of apoptotic cells has recently been implicated in disease pathogenesis.

 C1q deficiency, apoptosis and SLE

A possible explanation for this link has come from studies on C1q 'knock-out' mice who die of glomerulonephritis with the immunohistological features of human lupus. An increased frequency of apoptotic cells in their glomeruli suggests a role for C1q in the clearance of apoptotic cells.

The onset of disease is triggered by ultraviolet light, drugs and possibly infection. There is a plethora of immunological abnormalities, characterized by marked polyclonal B-cell activation associated with hypergamma-globulinaemia and production of autoantibodies.

Epidemiology

Systemic lupus erythematosus is nine times more common in women than in men. Onset is commonly in the second and third decades. Asians and black Americans are particularly susceptible.

 Factors responsible for exacerbations of SLE
- Exposure to sunlight (UV light)
- Psychological stress
- Infections
- Pregnancy and puerperium
- Drugs.

Characteristics of SLE
- Presence of numerous autoantibodies
- Circulating immune complexes
- Widespread tissue damage.

Clinical presentation

Many patients present with fever, arthralgia, fatigue and a skin rash. Additional features and major organ involvement (kidneys, CNS) may occur at disease onset or evolve. It has a long-term course characterized by exacerbations and remissions.

Musculoskeletal manifestations

Arthralgia is common (90%) but rarely progresses to deforming arthropathy. Hand deformities resulting from tendon disease may cause a rheumatoid-like non-erosive arthropathy (Jaccoud's arthropathy) in a minority of patients (Fig. 48).

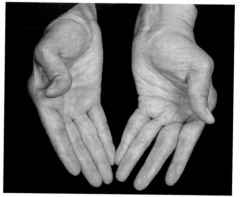

Fig. 48 Jaccoud's arthropathy in a patient with SLE.

Skin and mucous membranes

Ultraviolet light-induced skin photosensitivity is common. Malar rash and recurrent mouth ulcers occur in 50% of cases, non-scarring alopecia in 70% and Raynaud's phenomenon is a feature in 25%. Lupus confined to the skin is characterized by distinctive rashes—discoid lupus or subacute cutaneous lupus.

Kidney disease

Almost all patients with SLE have histological abnormalities on renal biopsy (see *Nephrology*, Section 1.9), but only 50% of patients develop overt renal disease.

Nervous system

Neurological involvement affects up to two-thirds of patients at some point in their disease (see Section 1.12, pp. 25–26).

Neuropsychiatric manifestations of SLE

Neuropsychiatric manifestations of SLE in decreasing order of frequency are:
- Organic brain syndrome—cognitive impairment, psychosis*
- Seizures
- Cranial neuropathy
- Peripheral neuropathy
- Cerebrovascular accident
- Movement disorder
- Transverse myelitis

*May be steroid induced.

Pulmonary

Pleurisy with or without radiological evidence of effusion occurs in 40% of cases. Acute lupus pneumonitis, fibrosing alveolitis and shrinking lung syndrome are rare manifestations in SLE.

Cardiovascular

Pericarditis (30%) is usually mild and very rarely progresses to tamponade. Non-infective thrombotic endocarditis (Libman–Sacks endocarditis) is rare and is associated with the antiphospholipid syndrome.

Haematological abnormalities

Normocytic normochromic anaemia and mild thrombocytopenia occur in a substantial number of patients. Reactive lymphadenopathy (40%) and splenomegaly (10%) occur especially during disease activity.

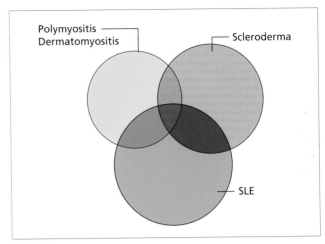

Fig. 49 Venn diagram depicting overlap of SLE, scleroderma and myositis.

The antiphospholipid syndrome occurs in 20% of patients with SLE.

Overlap syndromes

This term describes patients who have coexisting features of two or more connective tissue diseases (Fig. 49). The following are common examples:
- Scleroderma/SLE overlap
- Scleroderma/polymyositis overlap.

Mixed connective tissue disease

Patients with features of:
- SLE
- scleroderma
- polymyositis
were defined as having mixed connective tissue disease (MCTD) on the basis of high antibody titres to U1 ribonucleoprotein (U1 RNP), minimal renal disease and a good prognosis. The existence of MCTD as a distinct diagnostic entity has since been questioned because none of the clinical or laboratory criteria used for disease definition has proven specific.

Investigations

See Section 1.11, pp. 23–24.

Differential diagnosis

See Section 1.11, pp. 22–23.

Treatment

See Sections 1.11, p. 24 and 1.12, p. 26.

Prognosis

The 5-year survival rate is 90%, but at 15 years only 60% of patients with nephritis will be alive compared with 85% of those without nephritis. Mortality is caused by vasculitis, chronic renal failure, sepsis and cardiovascular complications.

2.4.2 SJÖGREN'S SYNDROME

 Sjögren's syndrome is a chronic autoimmune exocrinopathy predominantly affecting the salivary and lacrimal glands. The clinical picture is dominated by keratoconjunctivitis sicca (KCS) and xerostomia. It may occur by itself (primary Sjögren's syndrome) or in association with connective tissue disease (secondary Sjögren's syndrome) (Fig. 50).

Epidemiology

- Marked female preponderance
- M : F ratio 1 : 10
- Typically affects middle-aged women.

Aetiology/pathology

The cause of Sjögren's syndrome is unknown. Genetic markers include HLA-DR3, HLA-DQ2 and polymorphisms of the peptide transporter genes (*TAP-1*, *TAP-2*). An exhaustive search for a viral or environmental cause has proved to be fruitless. Epidemiological association with hepatitis C infection awaits confirmation. Inappropriate apoptosis has recently been implicated in disease initiation, while inhibition of apoptosis as a result of

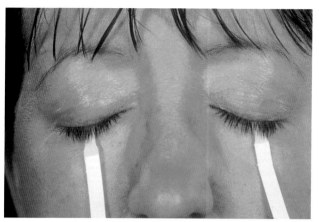

Fig. 51 Dry eyes in Sjögren's syndrome demonstrated by Schirmer's test: wetting of <5 mm of filter paper in 5 min is considered abnormal.

over-expression of the *bcl-2* oncogene has been implicated in the lymphoproliferation seen in established Sjögren's syndrome [2].

The cardinal pathological lesion is inflammatory destruction of salivary glands, mediated by focal periductular CD4+ T-cell infiltrates.

Clinical presentation

Keratoconjunctivitis sicca manifests as dry, gritty eyes (Fig. 51) on a background of fatigue. Poor salivary secretion leads to dysphagia for dry foods. Salivary gland enlargement (parotid and submandibular) occurs in 50% of cases.

 Other exocrine glands may be involved in Sjögren's syndrome. Impaired glandular function in the:
- nasal and sinus epithelium; and
- vagina

leads to recurrent sinusitis and dyspareunia, respectively.

Extraglandular features of Sjögren's syndrome
- Non-erosive arthritis
- Raynaud's phenomenon
- Cutaneous vasculitis
- Mixed cryoglobulinaemia
- Alveolitis
- Interstitial nephritis
- Risk of congenital heart block in babies of mothers with Sjögren's syndrome
- Mononeuritis multiplex.

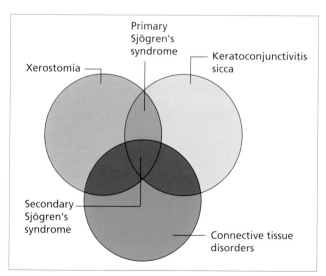

Fig. 50 Relationship between keratoconjunctivitis sicca, xerostomia, and primary and secondary Sjögren's syndrome. (Adapted with permission from Classification and assessment of rheumatic diseases. *Baillière's Clinical Rheumatology Journal* 1995; 9(3).)

Investigation

For laboratory findings, tests for KCS, the rose bengal test and tests for xerostomia, see Section 1.14, p. 29.

Treatment

See Section 1.14, p. 29.

Complications

There is an increased risk of B-cell lymphoma, estimated to be 33-fold in a recent Italian study [3].

Lymphoma in Sjögren's syndrome

Consider lymphoma if there is:
- persistent cervical lymph node enlargement
- persistent hard or nodular salivary or lacrimal gland enlargement
- lung shadowing
- monoclonal cryoglobulins
- progressive fall in serum immunoglobulins.

2.4.3 SYSTEMIC SCLEROSIS (SCLERODERMA)

Scleroderma is an autoimmune disorder characterized by excessive deposition of collagen. It leads to fibrosis and vascular obliteration within the skin and frequently within other organs, including the lung, heart, kidneys and gastro-intestinal tract.

Aetiology/immunopathogenesis

The aetiology is unknown. Despite wide-ranging immuno-logical activation it has been difficult to propose a single unifying immunopathogenic model. Several environmental agents (silica, organic solvents) have been implicated in disease initiation, but conclusive epidemiological evidence is lacking. The genetic component is exemplified by HLA associations (various HLA-DR alleles) with certain disease subsets. Recent interest has centred on the pos-sibility that microchimaerism as a result of persistence of fetal T cells in the mother might cause scleroderma by initiating a graft-versus-host response.

Key immunological features in scleroderma [4]
- Skin and lung lesions infiltrated by activated CD4+ and CD8+ T cells
- ↑ Expression of adhesion molecules from selectin, integrin and the Ig gene superfamily
- ↑ Production of TH_1 and TH_2 cytokines (IL1, IL2, IL4, IL6, IL8, TNF, TGFβ)
- Polyclonal B-cell activation leading to hypergammaglobulinaemia and autoantibody production.

Epidemiology

There is an annual incidence of 18 cases per 10^6 in the UK. The prevalence is estimated to be $100 : 10^6$. Female : male ratio is 3 : 1 and the incidence increases with age—it is most common at 30–50 years.

Table 26 Classification of scleroderma.

Disease extent	Features
Systemic	Diffuse cutaneous systemic sclerosis
	Limited cutaneous systemic sclerosis
	Systemic sclerosis *sine* scleroderma
	Overlap syndrome
Localized	Morphoea (localized, generalized)
	Linear scleroderma

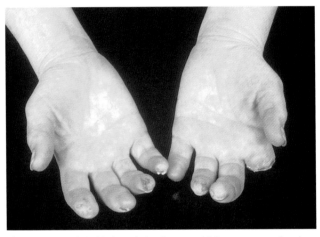

Fig. 52 Severe digital ischaemia leading to multiple autoamputations in a patient with diffuse cutaneous systemic sclerosis.

Clinical presentation

The classification of scleroderma is shown in Table 26.

Diffuse cutaneous scleroderma

The onset may be abrupt and may present as swollen hands (Fig. 52), face and feet associated with Raynaud's phenomenon. Fatigue is common and overt weakness may be present. Examination reveals inability to pinch skin folds, and loss of skin lines and creases in involved areas. Evaluation of swallowing, breathing, and renal and cardiac functions may reveal abnormalities.

Limited cutaneous systemic sclerosis

Limited systemic sclerosis was previously known as CREST (**c**alcinosis, **R**aynaud's, **o**esophageal dysfunction, **s**clerodactyly, **t**elangiectasia).

Typically the patient is a woman aged 30–50 with a long history of Raynaud's phenomenon and with recent skin involvement limited to the hands, face and feet (Table 27). Other features include the following:
- Calcium deposition in the skin (calcinosis) (Fig. 53)
- Dilated blood vessels (telangiectasia) in the palms and face
- Oesophageal dysmotility with or without reflux.

Table 27 Features helpful in differentiating diffuse systemic sclerosis (SS) from limited cutaneous disease.

	Diffuse cutaneous SS	Limited cutaneous SS
Extent of skin thickening	Truncal and acral	Acral
Timing of relationship between skin thickening and Raynaud's phenomenon	Simultaneous or skin first	Prolonged Raynaud's phenomenon before skin
Joints, tendon	Contractures, tendon friction rubs	Infrequent involvement
Calcinosis	Uncommon	Prominent
Visceral involvement	Renal, myocardial	Pulmonary hypertension
Serum autoantibodies	Anti-Scl 70 (30%)	Anticentromere (70%)

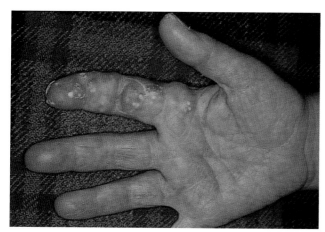

Fig. 53 Calcinosis cutis in the index finger of a patient with limited cutaneous systemic sclerosis.

Systemic sclerosis sine scleroderma

Some patients have visceral disease without cutaneous involvement. The presence of anticentromere, antiscleroderma-70 or antinucleolar antibodies is helpful in making the diagnosis.

Visceral involvement

Clinical spectrum of visceral involvement in scleroderma includes the following:
• Gastrointestinal tract: small mouth aperture and oesophageal hypomotility (90%). Malabsorption, wide-mouthed colonic diverticulae and rarely pneumatosis cystoides intestinalis.
• Lungs: pulmonary fibrosis, aspiration pneumonia, recur-rent chest infections, pleural thickening, effusion and calcifica-tion, spontaneous pneumothorax, pulmonary hypertension, pulmonary vasculitis and bronchoalveolar carcinoma.
• Cardiovascular system: pericarditis with effusion, myo-cardial fibrosis causing dysrhythmias and congestive cardiac failure.
• Kidney: hypertension, scleroderma renal crisis (acceler-ated hypertension) and progressive renal failure.

Investigations

Antinuclear antibodies

Antinuclear antibodies occur in 90% of patients. Three well-defined, mutually exclusive specificities have been defined (Fig. 54), each associated with certain clinical features and HLA alleles [5].

Hand radiograph

Loss of terminal phalangeal tufts and soft tissue calcifica-tion (calcinosis).

Visceral involvement

Assess extent of gastrointestinal involvement (manom-etry, endoscopy, contrast studies) and lung involvement (pulmonary function tests, high-resolution CT scans). Regular monitoring of blood pressure and renal function is essential in diffuse disease (risk of scleroderma renal

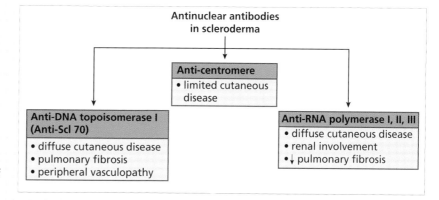

Fig. 54 Antinuclear antibodies in scleroderma allow for the definition of three mutually exclusive specificities.

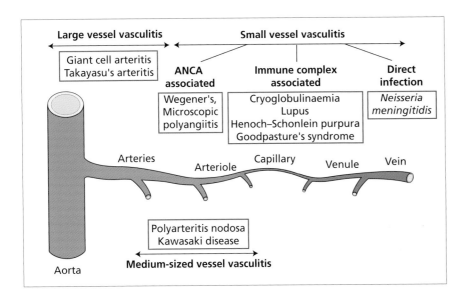

Fig. 55 Classification of vasculitides according to vessel size and underlying mechanisms. (Modified from Jennette JC, Falk RJ. Small vessel vasculitis. *N Engl J Med* 1997; 337: 1512–1523.)

crisis). Use Doppler echocardiography to detect pulmonary hypertension.

Treatment

Scleroderma is incurable. Treatment is aimed at the following:
- Alleviating the symptoms of Raynaud's phenomenon
- Preventing progression of lung fibrosis through the use of immunosuppressive therapy
- Controlling hypertension using ACE inhibitors
- Alleviating symptoms of reflux oesophagitis and gastrointestinal hypomotility.

Symptoms of Raynaud's phenomenon can be alleviated by stopping smoking, wearing thermal gloves, avoiding cold temperatures and prompt treatment of digital infections and ulcers. Oral vasodilators (Ca^{2+} channel blockers) are useful for frequent attacks. Prostacyclin infusions are useful in treating severe digital ischaemia.

Prognosis

The 5-year survival rate ranges from 30 to 70%. Adverse prognostic features include male sex, extent of skin involvement, and heart, lung and renal disease.

1 Mason LJ, Isenberg DA. Immunopathogenesis of SLE. *Baillière's Clin Rheumatol* 1998; 12: 385–403.
2 Humphreys-Beher MG, Peck AB, Dang H, Talal N. The role of apoptosis in the initiation of the autoimmune response in Sjögren's syndrome (editorial review). *Clin Exp Immunol* 1999; 116: 383–387.
3 Valesini G, Priori R, Bavoillot D *et al.* Differential risk of non-Hodgkin's lymphoma in Italian patients with primary Sjögren's syndrome. *J Rheumatol* 1997; 24: 2376–2380.
4 White B. Immunopathogenesis of systemic sclerosis. *Rheum Dis Clin North Am* 1996; 22: 695–708.
5 Harvey GR, McHugh NJ. Serologic abnormalities in systemic sclerosis. *Curr Opin Rheumatol* 1999; 11: 495–502.

2.5 Vasculitides

There is no single system of classification that would satisfy the heterogeneous group of vasculitides. In practical terms, it is best to classify the vasculitides using a combination of blood vessel size and underlying pathogenic mechanism(s), where these are known (Fig. 55).

2.5.1 GIANT CELL ARTERITIS AND POLYMYALGIA RHEUMATICA

Aetiology/pathophysiology/pathology

Giant cell arteritis (GCA) and polymyalgia rheumatica (PMR) are related disorders with common epidemiological, clinical and serological features [1]. Although GCA is a large-vessel vasculitis, PMR is a clinical syndrome characterized by prolonged proximal girdle pain and stiffness [2].

The aetiology of GCA and PMR is unknown. The clear preponderance of both disorders in elderly people remains unexplained. An increased frequency of HLA-DR4 and polymorphisms of the HLA-DRB1 genes suggests a genetic predisposition.

The cellular infiltrate in the synovium in PMR is very similar to the infiltrate found in the vascular lesions of GCA:
- CD68+ macrophages
- CD4+ T cells
- Giant cells.

A striking feature is the strong expression of HLA class II antigens on synovial and inflammatory cells. GCA affects all layers of the vessel wall, but is marked in the internal elastic lamina, where a granulomatous giant cell reaction is prominent. The thoracic aorta and its branches are commonly affected. Many of the characteristic clinical manifestations are the result of involvement of the branches of the external carotid artery.

Epidemiology

Ninety per cent of patients are >60 years age with a female pre-ponderance. GCA is the most common of the primary systemic vasculitides in white people (incidence $178 : 10^6$ population).

Clinical presentation

Common

Mild or severe headache occurs in two-thirds of patients often on a background of fatigue, fever and weight loss. PMR, with its characteristic proximal girdle pain and stiffness, occurs in 50% of patients with GCA and is the presenting feature in 25%. Claudication of the jaw muscles, producing pain on chewing, occurs in 40%, whereas visual symptoms resulting from ophthalmic artery involvement occur in 20% of patients.

Uncommon/rare

Occasionally, patients may present with pyrexia of unknown origin or dissecting aneurysms of the aorta.

Physical signs

Common

Scalp tenderness, frequently over the superficial temporal and occipital arteries, is highly suggestive of GCA and occurs in 40% of patients.

Uncommon

These include arterial bruits, asymmetrical blood pressure and absent pulses in extremities, and ophthalmoscopic evidence of ischaemic optic neuritis.

Investigations

There is no specific serological test. Elevated acute phase markers, in particular the ESR (>40 mm/h) and CRP, occur in 80% of patients and are useful indices for monitoring treatment. Arterial biopsy is recommended for diagnostic confirmation of GCA (Fig. 56) but, in practice, some clinicians reserve biopsy for patients who fail to respond to steroids. Arterial biopsy is not required in PMR, although it is positive in 10–20% of patients.

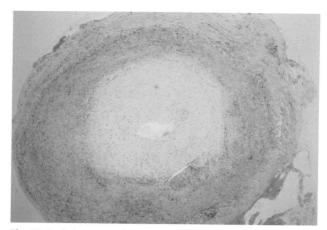

Fig. 56 Occluded temporal artery in a patient with giant cell arteritis showing thickening and lymphocytic infiltration throughout the vessel wall. (Courtesy of Dr L Bridges, Leeds General Infirmary.)

Differential diagnosis

A wide range of disorders may occasionally mimic PMR. Consider the alternative diagnoses listed in the key point below in cases of diagnostic doubt or failure to respond promptly to steroid therapy.

 Differential diagnosis of PMR

- Infection: tuberculosis, endocarditis
- Autoimmune rheumatic disease: rheumatoid arthritis, inflammatory muscle disease, systemic lupus
- Neoplasia
- Parkinsonism
- Hypothyroidism
- Chronic fatigue syndrome.

Treatment

Both GCA and PMR are exquisitely sensitive to steroids [3]. Indeed, failure to respond to steroids is sufficient cause for the original diagnosis to be questioned. The dose of steroids required to suppress inflammation is higher in GCA (40–60 mg/day); 10–20 mg is sufficient in PMR. The response to treatment is monitored using a combination of clinical and acute phase end-points (ESR, CRP). As most patients require treatment for 1–2 years it is essential to be alert to the problems of long-term corticosteroid therapy.

Complications

Permanent visual loss occurs in 15–20% of patients with GCA. A smaller percentage develop strokes and aortic aneurysms.

Prognosis

Overall prognosis for PMR is good, with 75% of patients stopping steroids by 2 years. Prognosis in GCA is determined by visual involvement (see above).

1 Hunder GG. Giant cell arteritis and polymyalgia rheumatica. *Med Clin North Am* 1997; 81: 195–219.
2 Salvarani C, Macchioni P, Boiardi L. Polymyalgia rheumatica (seminar). *Lancet* 1997; 350: 43–47.
3 Hayreh SS. Steroid therapy for visual loss in patients with giant cell arteritis. *Lancet* 2000; 355: 1572–1573.

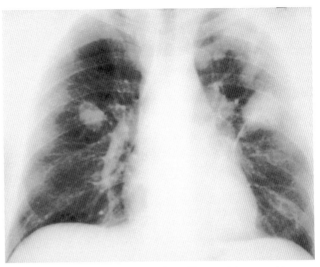

Fig. 57 Chest radiograph depicting bilateral lung nodules caused by pulmonary vasculitis in a patient with Wegener's granulomatosis.

2.5.2 WEGENER'S GRANULOMATOSIS

Aetiology/pathophysiology/pathology

Wegener's granulomatosis and microscopic polyangiitis (MPA) represent a spectrum of small vessel vasculitides associated with ANCAs (see *Nephrology,* Section 1.12).

The aetiology is unknown. Wegener's granulomatosis is characterized by necrotizing granulomatous vasculitis with little or no immune deposits [1]. Kidney biopsies typically show a pauci-immune glomerulonephritis.

Epidemiology

Wegener's granulomatosis affects both sexes equally. The peak incidence is in the fourth decade. The incidence of ANCA-associated vasculitis in the UK is estimated to be $20 : 10^6$ population per year.

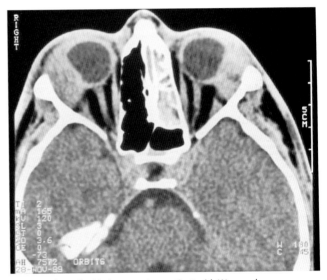

Fig. 58 Bilateral orbital masses in a patient with Wegener's granulomatosis. (Courtesy of Dr R Melsom, Bradford Royal Infirmary.)

Clinical presentation

Common

Most patients present with a pulmonary–renal syndrome (Fig. 57) on a background of upper respiratory tract involvement—haemoptysis, sinusitis, destruction of the nasal septum and epistaxis; 50% have ocular involvement in the form of conjunctivitis, scleritis and uveitis.

Uncommon

An uncommon presentation is cutaneous vasculitis with nail-fold infarcts and purpura.

Physical signs

Common

Despite the severity of systemic vasculitis, overt physical signs may be limited to a red eye in early disease. A collapsed nasal septum leading to a saddle nose is characteristic of established disease.

Uncommon/rare

• Proptosis caused by retro-orbital granulomas (Fig. 58)
• Cranial nerve deficits resulting from the spread of inflammation from the sinuses.

Table 28 Differential diagnosis of the pulmonary–renal syndrome.

Disorder	Key investigations
Wegener's granulomatosis/ microscopic polyangiitis	ANCA, histology
Goodpasture's syndrome	Antiglomerular basement membrane antibody, renal histology
Lupus	Antinuclear antibody, serum complement
Mixed cryoglobulinaemia	Cryoglobulin, rheumatoid factor, serum complement

Investigations

Antineutrophil cytoplasmic antibodies directed against proteinase-3 (PR3-ANCA) in high titre in this clinical setting are highly suggestive of Wegener's granulomatosis (see Section 3.2.5, p. 101). Histological confirmation of vasculitis on tissue biopsy (kidneys, nose or lung) is essential. Approximately 10% of patients are ANCA negative. Severity of inflammation is established by measuring serum CRP.

Differential diagnosis

The diagnosis is clear cut in patients presenting with ANCA-positive granulomatous vasculitis on a background of sinus, lung and kidney disease. Other disorders that present with a pulmonary–renal syndrome (Table 28) may occasionally pose problems.

Treatment

Emergency/short term

Combined treatment with steroids and cyclophosphamide induces remission in 90% of patients.

Long term

Maintain remission by continuing cyclophosphamide or alternative steroid-sparing agent (azathioprine, methotrexate) for 6–12 months. Fifty per cent of patients will relapse within 5 years. Note increased risk of bladder malignancy and acute leukaemia with long-term cyclophosphamide therapy [2].

 Be vigilant for infective problems (e.g. pneumocystis pneumonia) associated with long-term immunosuppression.

The role of co-trimoxazole in preventing infection-induced relapse is controversial.

 Consider use of intravenous immunoglobulin and therapeutic monoclonal antibodies (anti-CD52) in patients unresponsive to standard medication [3].

Complications

Common

- Chronic renal failure in 40%
- Collapsed nasal septum and subglottic stenosis in 30%
- Iatrogenic infertility in 50%.

Uncommon/rare

- Nasolacrimal duct obstruction.

Prognosis

The 5-year survival rate is >80%. This is largely determined by renal function at presentation. Significant long-term morbidity is caused by complications of the disease and its treatment (see above).

1 Hoffman GS, Kerr GS, Leavitt RY *et al.* Wegener's granulomatosis: an analysis of 158 patients. *Ann Intern Med* 1992; 116: 488–498.
2 Talar-Williams C, Hijazi YM, Walther MM *et al.* Cyclophosphamide induced cystitis and bladder cancer in patients with Wegener's granulomatosis. *Ann Intern Med* 1996; 124: 477–484.
3 Lockwood CM. Refractory Wegener's granulomatosis: a model for shorter immunotherapy of autoimmune diseases. *J R Coll Physicians Lond* 1998; 32: 473–478.

2.5.3 POLYARTERITIS NODOSA

Aetiology/pathophysiology/pathology

This is an immune complex-mediated vasculitis affecting medium-sized blood vessels.

The aetiology is unknown. It is associated with hepatitis B antigenaemia in 20%. Vasculitic lesions are triggered by deposition of immune complexes in endothelium with marked granulocytic infiltration of media, leading to aneurysmal dilatation.

Epidemiology

The peak incidence is in the fourth decade. The estimated annual incidence is $2.0–9.0 : 10^6$.

Clinical presentation

Common

Some 40–70% present with a purpuric or urticarial rash, myalgia, arthralgia and peripheral neuropathy, on a background of weight loss, hypertension and renal impairment.

Uncommon/rare

- Bowel perforation
- Orchitis
- Congestive heart failure.

Physical signs

Common

- Cutaneous signs (see above)
- 'Glove and stocking' sensory loss
- Mononeuritis multiplex
- Areflexia.

Uncommon/rare

- Testicular swelling
- Papilloedema
- Retinal detachment.

Investigations

The following are the key diagnostic investigations:
- Visceral/renal angiography to demonstrate aneurysms (Fig. 59)
- Tissue biopsy (muscle, sural nerve or kidney) for evidence of vasculitis.

Assess renal function and hepatitis B status. Use CRP to assess the severity of inflammation.

Differential diagnosis

Absence of glomerulonephritis and negative ANCA in PAN helps differentiate it from MPA. Consider the

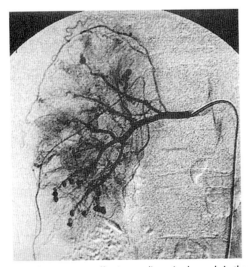

Fig. 59 Multiple aneurysms affecting medium-sized vessels in the right kidney in a patient with hepatitis B-associated polyarteritis nodosa. (With permission from Chauveau D, Christophe JL. Renal anevrysms in hepatitis B-associated polyarteritis nodosa. *N Engl J Med* 1995; 332: 1070.)

possibility of drug-induced vasculitis in young males, for example amphetamine or cocaine abuse may cause aneurysms.

Treatment

Systemic disease requires combined therapy with steroids and cyclophosphamide for about a year. Steroids alone are adequate for PAN confined to the skin.

Polyarteritis nodosa associated with hepatitis B is best treated with a combination of antiviral agents, i.e. vidarabine/lamivudine combined with interferon-α [1].

Complications

Common

- Chronic renal failure
- Hypertension.

Uncommon/rare

- Bowel infarction
- Acute bowel perforation.

Prognosis

Adverse prognostic factors causing increased mortality are: proteinuria >1 g/day, raised serum creatinine and visceral involvement [2]. The 5-year mortality rate in patients with all three factors is 46%.

1 Guillevin L. Treatment of classic polyarteritis nodosa in 1999. *Nephrol Dial Transplant* 1999; 14: 2077–2079.
2 Guillevin L, Lhote F, Gayraud M *et al.* Prognostic factors in polyarteritis nodosa and Churg–Strauss syndrome. *Medicine (Baltimore)* 1996; 75: 17–28.

2.5.4 CRYOGLOBULINAEMIC VASCULITIS

Aetiology/pathophysiology/pathology

This is an immune complex-mediated small-vessel vasculitis associated with mixed cryoglobulinaemia (MC), types II and III (see Table 9, p. 21). The precise reasons why immunoglobulins cryoprecipitate is not known. Of cases of MC, 60–80% are driven by underlying HCV infection [1]. Conversely, up to 50% of patients with HCV infection have a mixed cryoglobulinaemia [2], although only a small minority develop vasculitis.

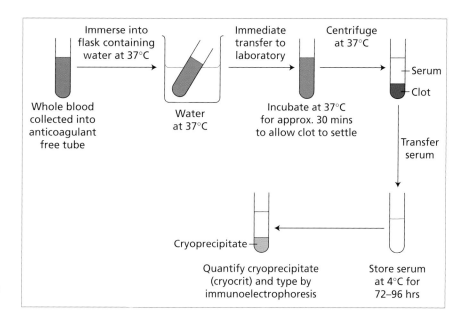

Fig. 60 Steps in the detection of cryoglobulins in the laboratory.

Type I cryoglobulins are associated with lymphoproliferative disease and rarely cause vasculitis.

Epidemiology

- Female preponderance
- Estimated incidence 1 : 100 000
- Higher incidence in southern Europe, reflecting prevalence of hepatitis C.

Clinical presentation

Common

- Triad of cutaneous vasculitis, glomerulonephritis and arthralgia (see Fig. 9, p. 21)
- Skin involvement occurs in almost all cases.

Uncommon/rare

- Mononeuritis multiplex
- Abdominal pain.

Physical signs

Common

- Purpuric skin rash
- Raynaud's phenomenon.

Uncommon/rare

- Sensory deficits
- Areflexia.

Investigations

 Important serological clues to the presence of mixed cryoglobulinaemia are a markedly low C4 and positive rheumatoid factor. Ensure that a blood sample for cryoglobulins is collected correctly at 37°C and transported immediately to the laboratory (Fig. 60).

Check hepatitis C serology, including hepatitis C RNA in the cyroprecipitate. Routine investigation for other infective triggers (endocarditis, syphilis, Lyme disease, malaria, HIV) reportedly associated with mixed cryoglobulinaemia is not warranted in the absence of suggestive clinical clues. Do a renal biopsy to assess renal damage.

Differential diagnosis

See Table 8, p. 20.

Treatment

See Section 1.10, p. 22.

Complications

Common

- Chronic renal failure in 50%
- Hypertension
- Leg ulcers.

Uncommon/rare

- Liver failure
- B-cell lymphoma.

Prognosis

The long-term outcome is determined by the extent of renal disease.

1 Ferri C, Zignego AL. Relation between infection and autoimmunity in mixed cryoglobulinaemia. *Curr Opin Rheumatol* 2000; 12: 53–60.
2 Wong VS, Egner W, Elsey T *et al.* Incidence, character and clinical relevance of mixed cryoglobulinaemia in patients with chronic hepatitis C virus infection. *Clin Exp Immunol* 1996; 104: 25–31.

2.5.5 BEHÇET'S DISEASE

Aetiology/pathophysiology/pathology

Behçet's disease is a syndrome of unknown aetiology, with vasculitis, hypercoagulability and neutrophil hyperfunction. It is diagnosed on clinical grounds, after the exclusion of similar diseases [1].

Epidemiology

It is most common in populations living along the 'Silk Road'—Japan, Korea and China to the Middle East and Turkey. The incidence and severity of disease are associated with HLA-B51 in these populations, but not in Westerners.

Clinical presentation

The disease typically presents with exacerbations and remissions.

Criteria for Behçet's disease

Defined by International Study Group for Behçet's disease [1]:
• Oral ulceration (at least three times per year).
• At least two of the following: genital ulceration (95% of cases), eye lesions (50–70% of cases), skin lesions (70–90% of cases), pathergy
• Absence of other diagnosis.

Common

Skin

• Erythema nodosum
• Vasculitic and acneiform lesions
• Superficial thrombophlebitis at venepuncture sites
• Pathergy: pustules at sites of skin puncture or minor trauma, such as bra straps (Fig. 61).

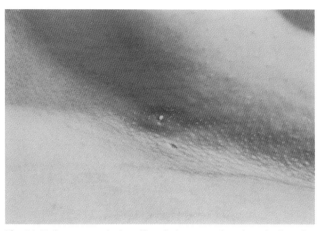

Fig. 61 Pathergy: pustular/acneiform lesions occurring along the line of the bra strap in a woman with Behçet's disease.

Eye

• Anterior or posterior uveitis: red, painful eye, loss of visual acuity, hypopyon
• Retinal vasculitis: loss of visual acuity.
Urgent ophthalmological opinion is necessary, even in patients who are asymptomatic, because uveitis and retinal vasculitis are common causes of blindness in Behçet's disease.

Joints

• Affected in 50–60% of cases
• Arthralgia or arthritis, usually large joints, non-erosive.

Uncommon

• Nervous system (10–20% of cases): cerebral vasculitis (transient ischaemic attacks, stroke, fits, progressive dementia, meningoencephalitis)
• Respiratory system: pulmonary vasculitis (episodes of dyspnoea, haemoptysis), pulmonary embolism
• Gastrointestinal system: intestinal vasculitis (abdominal pain, constipation, mesenteric angina, occasionally infarction with bloody diarrhoea)
• Cardiac: myocardial ischaemia or infarction.

Investigation

• ESR and CRP sometimes elevated in active disease
• Biopsies show vasculitis, with neutrophil infiltration of small and medium-sized vessels
• In cerebral disease, computed tomography is usually normal but MRI may show multiple high-signal white matter lesions (Fig. 62)
• Lumbar puncture may show raised protein, cells (lymphocytes, neutrophils) or neither.

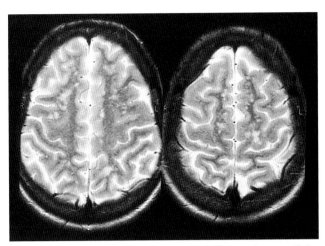

Fig. 62 MRI of the brain of a woman with Behçet's disease, who was suffering from transient ischaemic attacks. Note multiple high-signal lesions.

There is no diagnostic test—most investigations are for exclusion of other diseases. The presence of raised serum ACE, ANA, rheumatoid factor or ANCA should prompt you to consider an alternative diagnosis.

Differential diagnosis

- Herpes simplex (recurrent oral and genital lesions)
- Inflammatory bowel disease (gastrointestinal lesions)
- Multiple sclerosis (CNS lesions)
- Seronegative arthritis (arthritis and uveitis)
- Sarcoidosis (erythema nodosum, arthritis and uveitis)
- Sweet's syndrome (pathergy).

Treatment

 There are some remedies worse than the disease. (Publicus Syrus, 42 BC)

Behçet's disease is rare, and evidence for effectiveness of many of the standard treatments is lacking [2,3]. The following have been shown to be effective:
- Azathioprine and cyclosporin for eye disease
- Thalidomide for aphthous ulcers
- Benzathine–penicillin for joint disease.

High-dose steroids are used for initial control of acute severe exacerbations. In addition to the agents listed above, the following have been used for long-term treatment: cytotoxics (methotrexate, cyclophosphamide, chlorambucil), colchicine, interferon-α. Biological agents such as anti-CD52 or anti-CD18 have shown promise in small groups of patients.

 Whatever the therapy chosen, you will need to monitor clinical and laboratory indices for side effects. Remember that Behçet's disease is a relapsing–remitting disease and the patient may be able to enjoy periods of little or no drug therapy.

 • Methotrexate and thalidomide cause severe teratogenicity and are contraindicated in pregnancy, which must be avoided for at least 6 months after stopping methotrexate
• Cyclophosphamide and chlorambucil are teratogenic and may cause premature ovarian failure, particularly at high doses. These drugs are best avoided in a young female patient but, if considered essential, it is important that she is willing to use reliable contraception and to accept the risk of infertility.

Complications

Common

- Venous (including sagittal sinus) thrombosis and pulmonary embolism
- Pulmonary haemorrhage.

Venous thrombosis is common and presents a management dilemma because anticoagulation may precipitate life-threatening bleeding from vasculitic lesions. In practice most patients are anticoagulated without problems, although you would be wise to make a careful risk–benefit assessment and to distinguish pulmonary embolism from pulmonary vasculitis before commencing therapy.

Prognosis

This depends on the site and severity of disease. HLA-B51 is associated with a worse prognosis.

Morbidity

Blindness occurs in 25% of those with ocular lesions.

Mortality

Death is from thrombosis, haemorrhage or organ failure as a result of the vasculitis.

 1 Criteria for diagnosis of Behçet's disease. International Study Group for Behçet's Disease. *Lancet* 1990; 335: 1078–1080.
2 Sakane T, Takeno M, Noburu S, Inaba G. Behçet's disease. *N Engl J Med* 1999; 341: 1284–1291.
3 Saenz A, Ausejo M, Shea B *et al.* Pharmacotherapy for Behçet's syndrome. (Cochrane Review.) The Cochrane Library, 4, 2000, Oxford: Update Software.

2.5.6 TAKAYASU'S ARTERITIS

Aetiology/pathology

The cause of this arteritis is unknown; pathology of the arterial lesion is similar to that of giant cell arteritis, with focal granulomatous panarteritis associated with infiltration of CD4+ and CD8+ T cells. Fibrosis is a feature of advanced disease.

Epidemiology

It predominantly affects young females of Asian and South American origin [1]. The precise incidence rates in these countries are unknown. The annual incidence in the USA is $2.6 : 10^6$ population [2].

Clinical features

Early manifestations [1] include:
- malaise
- arthralgia
- myalgia
- elevated ESR.

Later in the course of disease, patients often present with claudication or hypertension, but few have inflammatory symptoms. Bruits and an absence of peripheral pulses are noted on physical examination (hence the term 'pulseless disease').

Pattern of disease

The disease primarily affects the aorta and its major branches (subclavian and carotid). A triphasic pattern of disease progression is seen:
- Stage I: pre-pulseless stage—fever, arthralgia and weight loss
- Stage II: vessel inflammation—vessel pain and tenderness (carotodynia).
- Stage III: burnt-out stage—bruits and ischaemia predominate.

Differential diagnosis

See Section 1.25, p. 52.

Investigation

See Section 1.25, pp. 52–53.

Treatment

See Section 1.25, p. 53.

Prognosis

For all patients, the 20-year survival rate is about 80%. In patients with one or more complications (retinopathy, hypertension, aortic valve disease, arterial aneurysms), this is reduced to 65%. Major causes of disability and/or mortality are heart failure, strokes and blindness.

1 Numano F. Differences in clinical presentation and outcome in different countries for Takayasu's arteritis. *Curr Opin Rheumatol* 1997; 9: 12–15.
2 Arend WP, Michel BA, Bloch DA *et al*. The American college of rheumatology 1990 criteria for the classification of Takayasu's arteritis. *Arthritis Rheum* 1990; 33: 1129–1134.

3 **Investigations and practical procedures**

3.1 Assessing acute phase response

3.1.1 ERYTHROCYTE SEDIMENTATION RATE

Principle

 The ESR, plasma viscosity (PV) and CRP are well-established markers of the acute phase response (APR) [1] (Tables 29 and 30).

The ESR is a measure of the rate of fall of red blood cells in a calibrated vertical tube.

 ESR measures the APR indirectly by reflecting changes in plasma proteins, particularly:
- fibrinogen
- α_2-macroglobulin
- immunoglobulins.

The ESR is also significantly influenced by changes in the number, shape and deformability of red blood cells, causing the ESR to rise with a fall in the haematocrit.

Indications

As it is influenced by plasma proteins of varying half-lives, the ESR represents, at best, a relatively crude way of assessing a persistent APR. The PV mirrors changes in the same plasma proteins that influence the ESR, but it is not altered by changes in haematocrit or red cell aggregability. For this reason and the ease of performing automated assays, there is an increasing tendency to substitute PV for ESR. However, the traditional role of both ESR

Table 29 Comparative utility of C-reactive protein (CRP), erythrocyte sedimentation rate (ESR) and plasma viscosity (PV) as markers of tissue damage I.

	CRP	ESR	PV
Change driven by	Cytokines: IL1, IL6, TNF Not dependent on changes in plasma proteins or red cells	Changes in plasma proteins and red cells	Changes in plasma proteins; unaffected by changes in red cells
Rapidity of change	↑ Within 6 h of onset of tissue damage; returns to normal within 48 h of resolution of inflammation/infection	↑ Within 24–48 h of onset of tissue damage; returns to normal over 4–6 days	Kinetics of response similar to ESR
Clinical utility	Highly sensitive and reproducible marker of inflammation, bacterial infection and tissue necrosis. Levels correlate with severity	Marker of chronic inflammation/infection Poor correlation with severity	As for ESR

Table 30 Comparative utility of CRP, ESR and PV as markers of tissue damage II.

	CRP	ESR	PV
Disorders characterized by major elevation	Inflammatory disease: RA, systemic vasculitis Infection: septicaemia, pyogenic abscesses	Systemic vasculitis Hyperglobulinaemic state: plasma cell dyscrasias, SLE, Sjögren's syndrome Systemic bacterial infection, e.g. infective endocarditis	As for ESR
Clinical situations associated with discordant responses	Raised ESR with normal CRP Consider: hyperglobulinaemia as in SLE, Sjögren's syndrome (without infection); anaemia, hyperlipidaemia		

and PV in monitoring chronic inflammatory disorders is being supplanted by CRP, a highly sensitive marker of the acute phase response.

3.1.2 C-REACTIVE PROTEIN

Principle

C-reactive protein is a member of the pentraxin family of proteins and is synthesized in the liver in response to proinflammatory cytokines (IL1, IL6 and TNF) during an acute phase response [2]. Circulating CRP is easily and accurately measured using nephelometry, a technique that measures the amount of light scattered by immune complexes of analyte (in this case CRP) and exogenous antibody. Given a constant antibody concentration, the amount of light scattered reflects the concentration of the analyte.

Indications

Its rapid rise within 6 h of the onset of tissue damage (peak at 48–72 h) makes CRP the most useful marker for monitoring inflammatory disease and systemic bacterial infection. Unlike the ESR or PV, CRP is not influenced by changes in plasma proteins or erythrocytes.

1 Ng T. Erythrocyte sedimentation rate, plasma viscosity and C-reactive protein in clinical practice. *Br J Hosp Med* 1999; 58: 521–523.
2 Pepys MB. The acute phase response and C-reactive protein. In: *Oxford Textbook of Medicine*, 3rd edn (Weatherall DJ, Ledingham JGG, Warrell DA, eds). Oxford: Oxford University Press, 1996: 1527–1533.

3.2 Serological investigation of autoimmune rheumatic disease

3.2.1 ANTIBODIES TO NUCLEAR ANTIGENS

Principle

Antibodies to nuclear antigens are detected by indirect immunofluorescence (IIF). Human epithelial cells (HEp-2) are used as source of antigen. HEp-2 cells are incubated with the patient's sera which contains autoantibodies. IgG antibodies reacting with antigens within the HEp-2 cells are recognized by adding a second anti-IgG antibody (conjugate) that contains a fluorochrome tagged to its Fc end (Fig. 63). Fluorescent microscopy is used to visualize the pattern of immunofluorescence produced by the autoantibody.

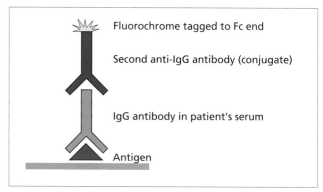

Fig. 63 Diagrammatic representation of indirect immunofluorescence for the detection of circulating antibodies.

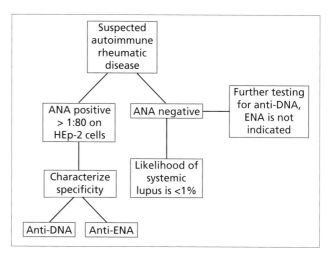

Fig. 64 Algorithm for the use of antibodies to nuclear antigens. ANA, antibodies to nuclear antigens; ENA, extractable nuclear antigens. (From Kavanaugh *et al.* Guidelines for clinical use of the antinuclear antibody test and tests for specific autoantibodies to nuclear antigens. *Arch Pathol Lab Med* 2000; 124: 71–81.)

Indications

Looking for ANA is the key initial investigation (Fig. 64) in patients with suspected SLE, lupus overlap disorders, Sjögren's syndrome and scleroderma (Table 31). Using HEp-2 cells as antigenic substrate, virtually all patients with untreated SLE are ANA positive.

 Previous reports of rare patients with ANA-negative lupus were based on studies using rodent tissue.

Antinuclear antibody is not specific for lupus and related disorders; it occurs in normal people and in a wide range of inflammatory and infective disorders.

Variants of ANA

Anticentromere antibodies

Antibodies directed against centromere antigens are

Table 31 Prevalence of autoantibodies in autoimmune rheumatic disease.

Disorder	ENA										
	ANA (%)	DNA (%)	Ro (%)	La (%)	Sm (%)	RNP (%)	ANCA (%)	Centromere(%)	Histones	Jo-1 (%)	Scl-70 (%)
SLE	99–100	60–90	35–60	Accompanies anti-Ro; rare in isolation	30	30–40	25 (p-ANCA)	Rare	50–70 of idiopathic SLE; 90–100 of drug-induced SLE	0	0
Scleroderma	60–90	0–5	0	0	0	0	NK	60	20	0	20–40
Primary Sjögren's syndrome	40–70	10	40–90	40–90	0	0	NK	Rare	NK	0	0
MCTD	100	0–5	0	0	0	100	NK	Rare	NK	Variable	Variable
Inflammatory myositis	40–70	0–5	0	0	0	0	NK	0	NK	30	0
Wegener's granulomatosis	? 5	0	0	0	0	0	80–95 (c-ANCA directed against PR-3)	0	NK	NK	0
Microscopic polyangiitis	? 5	0	0	0	0	0	≤80 (p-ANCA directed against MPO)		NK	NK	0

MCTD, mixed connective tissue disease; ENA, extractable nuclear antigens; ANCA, antineutrophil cytoplasmic antibody; NK, not known; PR3, proteinase-3; MPO, myeloperoxidase.

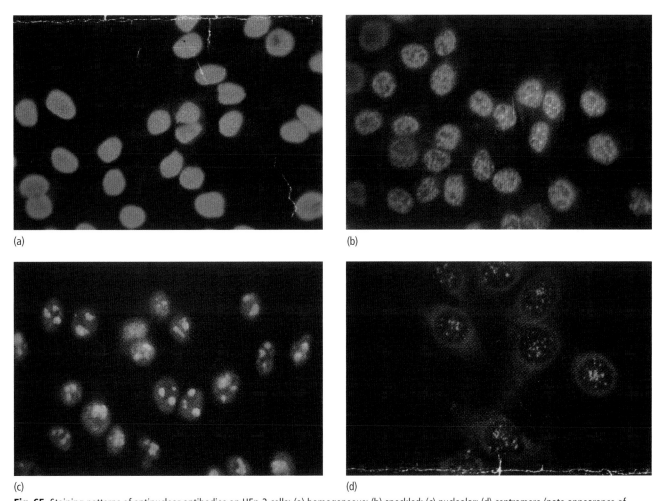

(a)

(b)

(c)

(d)

Fig. 65 Staining patterns of antinuclear antibodies on HEp-2 cells: (a) homogeneous; (b) speckled; (c) nucleolar; (d) centromere (note appearance of multiple fine dots representing staining of the kinetochores of 23 pairs of chromosomes). (Courtesy of Mr K Taylor, Leeds General Infirmary.)

easily detected by their characteristic pattern on HEp-2 cells by IIF (Fig. 65). Anticentromere antibodies are markers of the limited form of scleroderma, also known as the CREST syndrome (calcinosis, Raynaud's, oesophageal dysfunction, sclerodactyly, telangiectasia). Diffuse disease in scleroderma is associated with antibodies to the enzyme DNA topoisomerase (anti-Scl 70). Anti-Scl 70 is associated with more severe disease, especially pulmonary fibrosis.

Antihistone antibodies

Antibodies directed against histones, a group of highly conserved basic proteins in the nucleus, are associated with drug-induced lupus.

3.2.2 ANTIBODIES TO DOUBLE-STRANDED DNA

Principle

These are detected by a variety of techniques:
- Farr radioisotope assay
- Enzyme-linked immunoassay
- Indirect immunofluorescence using the haemoflagellate, *Crithidia luciliae* (Fig. 66).

In practice, enzyme-linked immunoassays are increasingly used in view of their high sensitivity, ease of automation and ability to quantify results reliably (Table 32).

Indications

A specific marker of SLE which is useful for the diagnosis and monitoring of disease activity in SLE. A steady rise in anti-DNA antibody levels heralds a lupus flare in many patients.

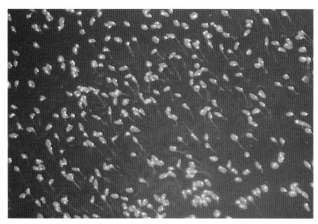

Fig. 66 Fluorescence confined to the kinetoplast of *C. luciliae* in a serum sample containing high concentrations of anti-DNA antibodies in a patient with active SLE.

Table 32 Comparison of three commonly used anti-double-stranded DNA assays in SLE.

	Farr	Crithidia	ELISA
Sensitivity	High	High	High
Specificity	High	High	Moderate
Detection of high avidity antibodies	+++	++	++
Detection of low avidity antibodies	+	++	+++
Ability to identify individual antibody isotypes (IgG, IgA, IgM)	No	Yes	Yes
Suitability for monitoring disease activity	Yes	No	Yes

ELISA, enzyme-linked immunosorbent assay.

3.2.3 ANTIBODIES TO EXTRACTABLE NUCLEAR ANTIGENS

Principle

 Extractable nuclear antigens refer to a group of saline-extractable antigens known individually as Ro, La, Sm and U1-RNP (uridine ribonuclear protein). Ro, La and Sm were named after the patients in whom they were first characterized: Robert, Lane and Smith. In conjunction with U1-RNP, these proteins are responsible for splicing and processing mRNA.

These antibodies are detected by a range of techniques:
- Immunoprecipitation assays such as countercurrent immunoelectrophoresis (CIE) or double diffusion
- Immunoblotting.

These techniques are specific, but are not suitable for handling large numbers of samples. Enzyme immunoassay is increasingly the method of choice but this may produce false-positive results in hypergammaglobulinaemic sera.

Indications

- Investigation of SLE
- Lupus overlap disorders
- Sjögren's syndrome.

Anti-Ro antibodies

Anti-Ro antibodies correlate with cutaneous disease and vasculitis in SLE. In pregnant women with lupus, anti-Ro antibodies may cross the placenta to cause transient cutaneous lupus in the neonate (5–25% of babies) or permanent congenital heart block (1–3% of babies). ANA-negative, anti-Ro-positive lupus is extremely rare (<1% of lupus patients). Consider primary complement deficiency in such patients. Anti-La antibodies tend to accompany anti-Ro ones.

Anti-Sm and U1-RNP antibodies

Anti-Sm antibodies are highly specific for SLE; their prevalence varies with the ethnic background of the patient. Anti-Sm and U1-RNP antibodies tend to occur together because of the shared peptide sequences between Sm and U1-RNP. The presence of anti-U1-RNP antibodies in isolation was thought to identify a group of patients with MCTD—a group of lupus overlap disorders with additional features of polymyositis and scleroderma. Long-term follow-up of the original cohort has raised questions about the existence of MCTD as a distinct entity.

3.2.4 RHEUMATOID FACTOR

Principle

Traditional sheep cell agglutination assays have been replaced by latex-enhanced turbidimetry or nephelometry (see Section 3.1.2).

Indications

- Prognostic marker in RA
- IgM rheumatoid factor occurs in 50–90% of patients with RA and in a wide range of other inflammatory and infective disorders.

3.2.5 ANTINEUTROPHIL CYTOPLASMIC ANTIBODY

Principle

Indirect immunofluorescence using human neutrophil as substrate is used to define patterns of ANCA. A cytoplasmic pattern of fluorescence (c-ANCA) is associated with antibodies directed against proteinase-3 (PR-3-ANCA), whereas a perinuclear pattern (p-ANCA) is associated predominantly with antibodies directed against myeloperoxidase (MPO-ANCA) (Fig. 67). Antigenic specificity is confirmed by enzyme immunoassay.

Indications

PR-3-ANCA and MPO-ANCA are sensitive markers of Wegener's granulomatosis and microscopic polyangiitis,

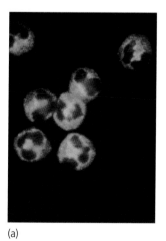
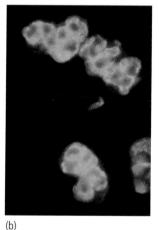

(a)   (b)

Fig. 67 Antineutrophil cytoplasmic antibodies (ANCAs): (a) granular cytoplasmic fluorescence with interlobular accentuation characteristic of c-ANCA; (b) perinuclear immunofluorescence characteristic of p-ANCA.

respectively. False positives may occur with infection, malignancy and other inflammatory disorders.

3.2.6 SERUM COMPLEMENT CONCENTRATIONS

Principle

C3 and C4 are assayed by nephelometry (see Section 3.1.2).

Indications

Indications are for the investigation of suspected systemic immune complex disease. Hypocomplementaemia is a characteristic feature of SLE and mixed cryoglobulinaemia, but it may also occur as a transient feature with infection, e.g. bacterial endocarditis.

> Kavanaugh A, Tomar R, Reveille J *et al.* Guidelines for clinical use of the antinuclear antibody test and tests for specific autoantibodies to nuclear antigens. *Arch Pathol Lab Med* 2000; 124: 71–81.
>
> Savige J, Davies D, Falk RJ *et al.* Antineutrophil cytoplasmic antibodies and associated diseases: a review of the clinical and laboratory features. *Kidney Int* 2000; 57: 846–862.

3.3 Suspected immune deficiency in adults

Principle

Immune deficiency

Suspect immune deficiency when:
- Infections are severe, frequent or prolonged
- Unusual (opportunistic) organisms are isolated
- In relatives of patients with known or suspected hereditary immunodeficiencies.

Antibody deficiency

Antibodies and complement are most important for extracellular organisms and for secondary protection against some viruses. Ask about the following:
- Bacterial infections
- *Giardia* spp.
- Enteroviruses.

Phagocyte defect

Phagocytes (neutrophils and macrophages) are scavengers, engulfing foreign material. They are important in the early response to infection (before the specific immune responses are under way) and, later, they are the effectors against organisms targeted by the specific immune response. Ask about the following:

• Septicaemia, periodontitis or deep abscesses with Gram-negative bacteria or staphylococci, invasive *Candida* or *Aspergillus* spp.
• Poor wound healing.

Screening for ciliary dysfunction

Ciliary dysfunction may masquerade as antibody deficiency. Test for this by placing a piece of saccharine tablet in the nose on the inferior turbinate. The patient should taste sweetness within 20 min if ciliary function is normal.

T-lymphocyte defect

T lymphocytes activate macrophages to kill organisms that they have phagocytosed, kill virus-infected cells and help B cells produce antibodies. Severe cellular defects present in infancy but milder forms may be diagnosed only in adulthood. Ask about the following:

• Viral infections: herpes simplex and zoster, cytomegalovirus, Kaposi's sarcoma, warts (including cervical intraepithelial neoplasia)
• Intracellular bacterial infections: salmonella infection, mycobacteria, including tuberculosis
• Mucocutaneous candidiasis
• Invasive cryptococci (meningitis)
• *Pneumocystis* sp. (pneumonia).
Consider secondary immunodeficiencies (Table 33).

Complement defects

An intact complement pathway is essential for the opsonization of micro-organisms and solubilization of immune complexes. Patients with terminal complement component deficiencies are prone to neisserial infection (see Sections 1.2, pp. 5–6 and 2.1.5, pp. 62–63), whereas early component deficiencies predispose to SLE.

Practical details

Detailed immunological investigations should be undertaken only in conjunction with an experienced clinical immunologist in order to ensure appropriate test selection.

Your investigations will depend on your clinical assessment. Your aim is to:

• define the immunodeficiency (if any); and
• assess your patient's individual risk of opportunistic infection, with a view to avoidance, prophylaxis or early treatment.

Basic investigations

For most patients, a sensible starting point would be to check the following:

• FBC and differential white cell count: lymphopenia is a feature of many cellular defects whereas a marked persistent neutrophilia (even in the absence of sepsis) would point to an adhesion molecule deficiency.
• Serum immunoglobulins as a basic screen of B-cell function. Exclude urinary loss of IgG by performing urine electrophoresis in patients with an isolated low IgG.
• Lymphocyte surface markers (e.g. CD3, -4, -8 for total, helper and cytotoxic T cells; CD19 for B cells; CD16 for natural killer [NK] cells) to quantify numbers of circulating lymphocytes. Close liaison with the clinical immunology laboratory is essential for selection of appropriate markers.

Antibody deficiency

Diagnosing antibody deficiency is relatively straightforward in patients with marked hypogammaglobulinaemia. If serum immunoglobulins are normal or moderately low, or there is isolated IgA deficiency, check baseline antibody levels to common pathogens (*Strep. pneumoniae*) and routine immunizations (tetanus, diphtheria, *Haemophilus influenzae* type b).

Cause	Deficiency
Drugs	
Steroids and cytotoxics	Cellular deficiency or neutropenia (quantitative/functional)
Antiepileptics	Antibody deficiency
Penicillamine, gold	
Carbimazole	Idiopathic neutropenia
Antibiotics	Disruption of normal bacterial flora
Smoking	Impaired mucociliary clearance
Viral respiratory tract infections	Impaired mucociliary clearance
HIV	Cellular deficiency
Haematological malignancy	Cellular, antibody or complement deficiency
Burns, wounds (skin), severe eczema	Breach of protective barrier

Table 33 Common causes of secondary immunodeficiency.

A normal serum immunoglobulin profile does not exclude significant antibody deficiency.

If antibody levels are low, proceed to test immunization with appropriate killed vaccines or toxoid (tetanus toxoid, Pneumovax, *Haemophilus influenzae* type b conjugate [Hib]) and recheck antibody levels 3–4 weeks later. IgG subclass measurements are of limited value and are meaningless without information about the specific antibody production.

 Live vaccines should be avoided in suspected immunodeficiency because of the risk of vaccine-induced disease, e.g. paralytic poliomyelitis caused by oral polio vaccine.

Establishing the cause

 Severe hypogammaglobulinaemia accompanied by lack of circulating B cells is suggestive of a defect in B-cell differentiation.

If B cells are absent consider checking for mutations in the following:
- Bruton tyrosine kinase gene (X-linked)
- μ heavy chain gene (autosomal recessive)
- λ5 light chain gene (autosomal recessive)
- Igα (CD79a) gene, a component of the pre-B cell receptor.

In male patients with hypogammaglobulinaemia and a normal or high serum IgM, exclude CD40 ligand deficiency.

Complement deficiency

Check integrity of complement pathways by checking haemolytic activity of the classic and alternate pathways (CH50 and AP50) (see Section 2.1.5, p. 62).

Consider secondary causes: C3 nephritic factor, an IgG autoantibody that stabilizes the alternate pathway C3 convertase causing consumption of C3 (associated with mesangiocapillary glomerulonephritis); immune complex disease.

T-lymphocyte defect

Total lymphocyte and individual lymphocyte subset numbers are usually low. Check additionally for HLA class I and II expression by flow cytometry. Check lymphocyte proliferation to mitogen (stimulates all lymphocytes), such as PHA, and antigen (stimulates only lymphocytes with appropriate T-cell receptor), such as PPD or tetanus

toxoid. Consider in vivo intradermal testing to a range of antigens (PPD, *Candida* spp., tetanus, streptokinase).

Establishing the underlying causes

Delineate aetiology in appropriate cases by the following:
- Chromosomal analysis (22q11 associated with absent thymus)
- Enzyme assays (adenosine deaminase and purine nucleoside phosphorylase [PNP] deficiency is associated with progressive combined deficiencies).

 A useful clue to PNP deficiency is the presence of marked hypouricaemia, reflecting the key role of PNP in urate production.

Phagocyte defect

Check for cyclical neutropenia. Do neutrophil counts three times weekly for 1 month. Do an NBT test (see Fig. 6, p. 12).

Check for leucocyte adhesion defects: flow cytometry to check for presence of adhesion molecules, especially CD18. Assess neutrophil chemotaxis.

Determining risk of infection

Knowledge of the patient's individual immune defect, combined with his or her probable exposure to pathogens, will help determine the likelihood of infection (Table 34). Take a thorough history, including travel and immunization history. Serological tests based on antibody detection are likely to be unreliable in the presence of immunodeficiency, but may give information about previous exposure (risk of reactivation) or immunity (risk of severe disease if non-immune). Cultures, biopsy and antigen-detection techniques (immunofluoresence or PCR) will usually be necessary to diagnose active infections, because clinical features may be atypical in immunodeficient individuals. Invasive investigations may be required.

 Chapel H, Webster D. Assessment of the immune system. In: *Primary Immunodeficiency Diseases. A molecular and genetic approach* (Ochs HD, Smith CIE, Puck JM, eds). Oxford: Oxford University Press, 1998.

Conley ME, Notarangelo LD, Etzioni A. Diagnostic criteria for primary immunodeficiencies. *Clin Immunol* 1999; 93: 190–197.

Fischer AJ, Cavazzana-Calzo M, de Saint Basile G et al. Naturally occurring primary deficiencies of the immune system. *Annu Rev Immunol* 1997; 15: 93–124.

	Antibody/complement	Cell mediated	Phagocyte
Bacterial	*Streptococcus pneumoniae*	*Salmonella* spp.	*Staphylococcus aureus* and *Staph. epidermis*
	Haemophilus influenzae	*Listeria* spp.	*Escherichia coli*
	Neisseria meningitidis	*Nocardia* spp.	*Klebsiella* spp.
	Mycoplasma spp.	Mycobacteria (TB, aytpical)	*Pseudomonas* spp.
Viral	Enteroviruses; including invasive echovirus and polio*	Herpes viruses; including HSV-1 and -2, invasive CMV, lymphomas (EBV) and Kaposi's sarcoma (HHV8) Papilloma virus (warts, cervical and anal neoplasia) JC virus (progressive multifocal leucoencephalopathy)	
Fungal		*Candida* spp. (mucocutaneous) *Pneumocystis* spp. Cryptococci	*Candida* spp. (invasive), *Aspergillus* spp.
Protozoal	*Giardia* spp.*	*Toxoplasma* spp. *Cryptosporidium* spp., *Microsporidium* spp.	

Table 34 Patterns of infection in immunodeficiency.

CMV, cytomegalovirus; EBV, Epstein–Barr virus; HHV, human herpes virus; HSV, herpes simplex virus.
* Giardia and enteroviral infections are not a feature of complement deficiency.

3.4 Imaging in rheumatological disease

3.4.1 PLAIN RADIOGRAPHY

Principle

The primary use of radiography is to detect changes in bony structure. It is much less useful in soft-tissue pathology.

Indications

Diagnostic

• Differential diagnosis of chronic arthritis: inflammatory, erosive arthritis can be distinguished from OA. Distinct forms of inflammatory arthritis can be further differentiated (Fig. 68).
• Back pain: plain radiographs are greatly overused in the assessment of back pain. However, in 'red flag' back pain (see Section 1.17, p. 34), plain radiographs may provide definitive diagnostic information (e.g. osteoporotic fracture, ankylosing spondylitis) or provide pointers to appropriate further investigation (e.g. in suspected malignancy or septic discitis). Plain radiographs hardly ever help in the assessment of neurological problems.
• Metabolic bone disease: diagnostic in Paget's disease, supportive in osteomalacia, unhelpful in osteoporosis (unless fracture present).

• Malignancy: few definitive diagnostic findings, but often strong supportive evidence in both primary and metastatic bone tumours.

Prognosis/disease outcome

Plain radiographs play a major role in assessing progress of inflammatory arthritis. The development of bony erosions, the progression of erosive changes and the development of secondary osteoarthritic changes are the most robust methods for assessing articular damage, prognosis and response to treatment (see Sections 1.19, pp. 39–41 and 2.3.3, pp. 72–75).

In RA, annual or biannual serial radiographs of the hands (Fig. 69) and wrists are the most useful means of monitoring the rate of joint damage and assessing the effects of treatment. Early development of erosions is one of the best predictors of aggressive disease. Radiographs of larger joints in RA are only useful in documenting the development of secondary OA. Neck pain or neurological signs in the limbs should provoke a radiograph of the cervical spine, particularly to look for atlantoaxial subluxation. Views in cervical flexion and extension are required.

> **Limitations of plain radiographs**
>
> • Radiation exposure
> • Failure to detect soft-tissue pathology
> • Changes only appear late in the disease process; neoplastic and inflammatory bone destruction is usually well advanced before it is evident on a plain film.

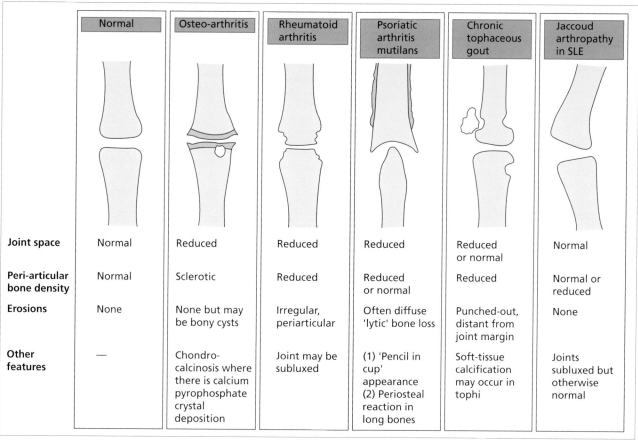

	Normal	Osteo-arthritis	Rheumatoid arthritis	Psoriatic arthritis mutilans	Chronic tophaceous gout	Jaccoud arthropathy in SLE
Joint space	Normal	Reduced	Reduced	Reduced	Reduced or normal	Normal
Peri-articular bone density	Normal	Sclerotic	Reduced	Reduced or normal	Reduced	Normal or reduced
Erosions	None	None but may be bony cysts	Irregular, periarticular	Often diffuse 'lytic' bone loss	Punched-out, distant from joint margin	None
Other features	—	Chondro-calcinosis where there is calcium pyrophosphate crystal deposition	Joint may be subluxed	(1) 'Pencil in cup' appearance (2) Periosteal reaction in long bones	Soft-tissue calcification may occur in tophi	Joints subluxed but otherwise normal

Fig. 68 Schematic representation of radiological changes in major arthritides. These changes are found in advanced, long-standing disease. Radiographs may be normal in early disease.

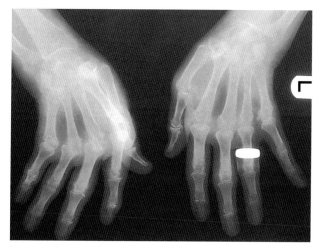

Fig. 69 Radiograph of the hands in a patient with advanced rheumatoid arthritis showing deforming, erosive arthropathy.

3.4.2 BONE DENSITOMETRY

Principal

Plain radiographs cannot provide a reliable assessment of bone mineral density (BMD). Several techniques exist for quantitating absorption of radiation by bone, while compensating for absorption by soft tissues. Dual-energy X-ray absorptiometry (DEXA) scanning is the most widely used technique, because it is highly accurate and involves low radiation exposure. BMD is usually measured at the hip and lumbar spine and results expressed as the following:

• Standard deviations above (+) or below (−) the mean for the patient's sex and age (Z score)
• Standard deviation from the mean BMD for a young adult (T score).

Fracture risk varies continuously with reduction in BMD and approximately doubles with each standard deviation below the mean. However, osteoporosis is usually defined as BMD T score <−2.5.

Indications

BMD measurement should be used only where the result will influence treatment. If a decision has been made to treat on clinical grounds (e.g. with hormone replacement therapy in a woman with an early menopause, maternal history of hip fracture and a vertebral crush fracture), then DEXA scanning is unlikely to add anything useful.

When to use DEXA

DEXA scanning should be considered in the following circumstances:
- Plain radiographs suggest osteopenia or vertebral deformity
- Previous fragility fractures have occurred
- Prednisolone therapy (or equivalent other corticosteroids) for >6 months at doses >7.5 mg
- Gonadal failure (early menopause, prolonged amenorrhoea, hypogonadism in men)
- Chronic systemic ill-health, especially if weight loss, malabsorption or metabolic bone disease
- Serial monitoring of BMD in response to treatment or risk factors such as corticosteroid treatment.

3.4.3 MAGNETIC RESONANCE IMAGING

Principle

Magnetic resonance imaging utilizes the changes in magnetic field induced by excitation of hydrogen protons to produce cross-sectional imaging; these can powerfully differentiate types of soft tissue, largely on the basis of water content. Cross-sectional images can be constructed in any plane. Scans are usually performed to detect two different patterns of change in magnetic field, known as T1-weighted (T1w) and T2-weighted (T2w) scans. T1w scans show high signal from fat, but not fluid, whereas T2w scans show both fat and fluid as high signal. The signal from fat can be suppressed from a T2w scan to give selective imaging of the fluid content.

Tissues with a low fluid and fat content (e.g. bone, ligament and tendon) appear dark on MRI, whereas pathological processes such as inflammation or neoplasia appear bright on T2w scans because of their rich blood supply.

Indications

MRI is an extremely sensitive technique. Minor pathology of doubtful significance is frequently demonstrated, e.g. scans of the lumbar spine are rarely 'normal' over the age of 40. Great care needs to be exercised when requesting and interpreting MRI scans. Scans performed as a 'screening' exercise, without a sound diagnostic hypothesis, are more likely to confuse than to inform.

When to use MRI

MRI may provide diagnostic information in the following:
- Red flag pattern back pain: suspected malignancy, discitis or serious neurological involvement (see Section 1.17, p. 34)
- Cervical and lumbar pain with neurological involvement: particularly spinal cord pathology
- CNS disease in systemic lupus or systemic vasculitis

When to use MRI (*continued*)
- Suspected avascular necrosis of bone: changes may predate plain radiographs by several weeks; surgical intervention is unlikely to be helpful once changes are seen on a plain radiograph
- Polymyositis: useful in patchy disease, both diagnostically and to identify sites for biopsy
- Mechanical knee pain: as useful as arthroscopy in demonstrating meniscal or ligament pathology
- Shoulder pain: assessment of the rotator cuff
- Suspected soft-tissue tumours: malignant and benign tumours can usually be distinguished, and pointers to histology can be found (e.g. haemangioma, neurofibroma, lipoma, synovial cyst)
- MRI of inflammatory arthritis can be used to detect synovitis and early erosive changes, but currently it is largely a research tool.

Contraindications

MRI is free from radiation hazards, although scanning in the presence of mobile pieces of metal in anatomically fragile sites can have disastrous consequences—intracranial aneurysm clips, foreign bodies in the eye and permanent pacemakers all rule out MRI. Imaging can be performed with fixed non-mobile metal such as joint prostheses, although the quality of imaging may be poor near the metal object.

3.4.4 NUCLEAR MEDICINE

Principle

A short-lived radioisotope that emits gamma radiation is tagged on to either a pharmacologically active molecule or whole cells. After injection, the localization of the isotope is visualized with a gamma camera. In general, scintigraphic techniques are strong at providing information on function, but relatively weak on anatomical definition. Radioisotope bone scanning is the most commonly used technique in rheumatology: this utilizes technetium-99m-labelled bisphosphonates, which are taken up at sites of bone turnover.

Indications

Bone scintigraphy

- Suspected stress fracture: scintigraphic changes may predate plain radiograph changes by 2 or more weeks
- Suspected osteomyelitis: again, scintigraphy precedes plain radiograph changes
- Metabolic bone disease: may strongly support diagnosis of Paget's disease (Fig. 70) or osteomalacia
- Peripheral joint disease: limited utility in defining distribution of an arthritic process
- Suspected bony malignancy: sensitive but low specificity.

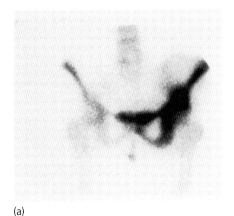

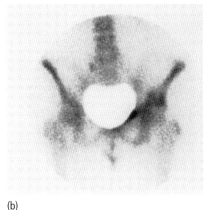

Fig. 70 Isotope bone scan showing Paget's disease of the pelvis (a) before and (b) after treatment with pamidronate infusions.

(a)

(b)

 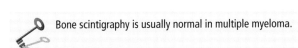

Bone scintigraphy is usually normal in multiple myeloma.

Inflammation or infection

This is most commonly performed using radiolabelled autologous leucocytes. This is of particular use in locating occult sepsis (e.g. in pyrexia of unknown origin).

Amyloid

The diagnosis and response to treatment of all forms of amyloidosis is facilitated by scintigraphy, using radiolabelled serum amyloid P protein. Unfortunately this technique is restricted to a small number of centres.

Maddison PJ, Isenberg DA, Woo P, Glass DN (eds). *Oxford Textbook of Rheumatology*, 2nd edn. Oxford: Oxford University Press, 1998. Section 4.9. (A useful overview.)
Resnick D. *Diagnosis of Bone and Joint Disorders.* Philadelphia: WB Saunders, 1995. Comprehensive reference work.

3.5 Arthrocentesis

Principle

Aspiration of synovial fluid is the most useful diagnostic manoeuvre in the differential diagnosis of joint disease (see Section 1.18, pp. 37–38). Macroscopic examination of synovial fluid may demonstrate the clear, viscous synovial fluid found in osteoarthritis and other non-inflammatory disorders, and the turbid fluid of inflammatory arthritis or haemarthrosis. The use of Gram stain, culture and polarized light microscopy will differentiate septic arthritis, crystal arthritis and other inflammatory arthritides. Some specialized laboratories may be able to differentiate between different forms of inflammatory arthritis on the basis of the differential cell count and other cytological features.

Indications

• Any inflammatory arthritis or joint effusion of uncertain cause
• Any established inflammatory arthritis that behaves in an unexpected fashion (e.g. a severe monoarticular flare in otherwise stable rheumatoid disease—this may be the result of septic arthritis).
Lack of experience in the technique is not an excuse—if you can't do it, find someone who can!

Contraindications

There are very few contraindications:
• Probable periarticular sepsis (e.g. cellulitis overlying a inflamed joint) may lead to introduction of sepsis into the joint.
• Prosthetic joints should usually be left to the orthopaedic surgeons.
• Warfarin treatment with INR in the therapeutic range is not a contraindication, but severe bleeding tendencies (e.g. severe haemophilia or thrombocytopenia severe enough to cause spontaneous bleeding) should usually be corrected before aspiration.

 Prosthetic joint problems should be referred to the orthopaedic surgeons. Never aspirate a prosthetic joint without at least discussing this with your orthopaedic colleagues.

Practical details

Before the procedure

Arthrocentesis can be performed in the outpatient clinic or at the bedside. No equipment is needed other than something to clean the skin and a needle and syringe. In general use a green 21 G needle for large joints such as the knee or shoulder, and a blue or orange needle for smaller joints. Use of too small a needle may prevent aspiration of viscous fluid.

Most rheumatologists use a 'no-touch' technique, whereby the site of aspiration is identified and often marked before skin preparation and aspiration is then performed without the use of sterile gloves. If gloves are not used, the hands should be washed carefully.

Choose a size of syringe appropriate to the size of the effusion—you are unlikely to aspirate more than 1–2 mL from the wrist, but an acutely swollen knee may contain >200 mL of fluid.

Most experienced aspirators do not use local anaesthetic to the skin and soft tissues, because infiltration of local anaesthetic can be as uncomfortable as the procedure itself.

The less experienced in joint aspiration may prefer to use sterile gloves and local anaesthetic because this allows the position of the needle to be checked with respect to the joint margins, and allows for some hesitancy in the advance of the needle.

The procedure

Detailed instructions for individual joints cannot be given here. However some general points apply:

1 Palpate the inflamed joint
2 Decide whether a fluctuant effusion is present
3 Mark the point of entry and clean the skin with alcohol or iodine
4 Insert the needle at the point of maximum fluctuation, taking care to avoid major neurovascular structures (e.g. the ulnar nerve at the elbow)
5 Entry to the joint cavity will usually be with a palpable 'give'
6 Draw back on the syringe at intervals as the needle is advanced until fluid is obtained
7 Aspirate as much fluid as possible without causing undue discomfort
8 If no obvious effusion is present, fluid is less likely to be obtained. However, in some deep-seated joints such as the hip, shoulder and elbow, significant effusions may be present even when not palpable at the surface.

Virtually all extraspinal joints can be aspirated at the bedside, guided by surface anatomy. The exception is the hip, which is so deep seated that aspiration under radiological or ultrasonic control is recommended. Radiological help can also be invaluable with effusions that are difficult to aspirate but clinically important.

After the procedure

Samples for microbiological examination should be placed in a clean sterile container. Some laboratories prefer an anticoagulant sample for polarized light microscopy and cytology—check with your local lab first. Samples should arrive at the laboratory within the same working day, although samples stored overnight may be suitable for culture and detection of crystals. (See Sections 1.18, p. 38, 2.3.6, p. 81 and 2.3.7, p. 82.)

Diagnostic microscopy and culture can be performed on less than 0.5 mL, and crystals can sometimes be seen in the flushings from the needle of an apparently dry tap, so it may be worth taking the needle and syringe to the laboratory.

Complications

Complications are rare:
• Major: infection may rarely be introduced into the joint; the risk is less than 1 : 30 000.
• Minor: some discomfort is inevitable but this is usually minor.

All of the large rheumatology textbooks contain comprehensive illustrated descriptions of joint aspiration and injection techniques, especially *Oxford Textbook of Rheumatology*, 2nd edn, 1998.
Freemont AJ, Denton J. *Atlas of Synovial Fluid Cytopathology*. Dordrecht: Kluwer Academic, 1992. Gives a detailed account of all aspects of synovial fluid microscopy.

3.6 Corticosteroid injection techniques

Principle

A suspension of poorly soluble corticosteroid crystals is injected into an inflamed joint or soft-tissue lesion. This produces a prolonged, potent, local anti-inflammatory effect with minimal systemic corticosteroid action.

Indications

This technique is one of the most useful therapeutic manoeuvres in rheumatology and is useful in the following:
• Non-septic inflammatory arthritis in any joint
• Selected cases of non-inflammatory arthritis
• Soft-tissue rheumatic disorders: tennis elbow, plantar fasciitis, trochanteric bursitis
• Carpal tunnel syndrome, especially when resulting from an inflammatory cause.

Contraindications

Absolute

- Septic or suspected septic arthritis
- Septicaemia
- Allergy to any component of the corticosteroid preparation
- Prosthetic joints
- Infected skin overlying joint.

Relative

- Peritendinous injection may predispose to subsequent rupture of the tendon, especially the Achilles' tendon and the long head of biceps. Injection at these sites should be at the discretion of a senior colleague.
- Bleeding tendency.

Practical details

The preparation and techniques for introduction of a needle into a joint (Figs 71 and 72) are described in Section 3.5, pp. 107–108. Aspiration of the joint before injection is not always required (if you don't know the diagnosis, you shouldn't be injecting) and may not be possible if no effusion is present. However, large or tense effusions should be aspirated because this will make the joint less uncomfortable. Some rheumatologists recommend that any fluid that can be aspirated should be sent for culture, to exclude unrecognized infection.

If aspiration is being performed before injection, the syringe for aspiration should be removed, leaving the needle *in situ*, and the syringe containing the corticosteroid preparation carefully placed in the hub of the needle, taking care not to touch any sterile area. Even if aspiration is not

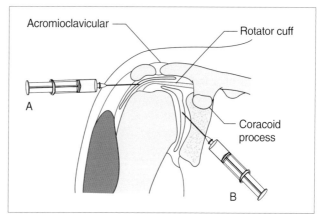

Fig. 72 Injection of the (A) subdeltoid and (B) glenohumeral joint. (With permission from the Arthritis and Rheumatism Council.)

performed before injection, the gentle suction should be placed on the aspirating syringe as you enter the joint—reflux of synovial fluid confirms that you are in the joint space.

> **!**
> - Injection into the joint space should meet almost no resistance and be almost pain free
> - Accurate intra-articular placement gives a better response than periarticular injection.

Individual soft-tissue injection techniques cannot be described here. In general, the corticosteroid is injected directly at the site of pathology, into the most tender area. Soft-tissue injections are therefore usually more painful than intra-articular injections.

The steroid preparations used most commonly are poorly soluble salts of methylprednisolone, triamcinolone and hydrocortisone. Hydrocortisone preparations are the least potent and shortest acting, and are often preferred for use in superficial soft-tissue or peritendinous injections to reduce the risk of skin atrophy and tendon rupture. The differences between the other preparations are not great. The amount of steroid injected depends on the size of the joint, e.g. 40–80 mg (1–2 mL) methylprednisolone is appropriate for a large joint such as a knee, but only 5–10 mg (0.25–0.5 mL) for a small finger joint.

Many rheumatologists use a mixture of steroids and local anaesthetic for injection. The evidence for any beneficial effect of local anaesthetic mixtures is small, but they may reduce discomfort after injection, particularly for soft-tissue injections. Only methylprednisolone and lidocaine (lignocaine) are available in a premixed form.

In theory, any number of joints may be injected in a single session, but in practice this is limited by discomfort and the cumulative dose of steroids. In practice, it is recommended that no more than three or four joints are injected in one session.

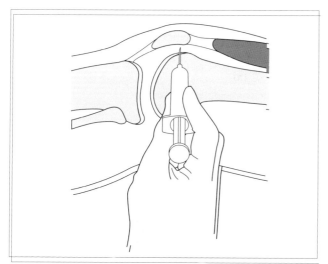

Fig. 71 Injection of the knee joint in extension. (With permission from the Arthritis and Rheumatism Council.)

Outcome

Improvement usually occurs within 24–48 h. Historically, most rheumatologists recommended 24–48 h bed rest after injection of a weight-bearing joint, but this is no longer practical or necessary. Advice to minimize weight bearing of the affected joint does, however, seem to be associated with a modest increase in efficacy.

 The duration of response after injection depends on the severity of synovitis, although improvement is usually for weeks to months. A rapid relapse of inflammation in a patient with a chronic arthritis should lead you, first, to question the diagnosis (could this be sepsis?) and, second, to question whether the patient's systemic medication needs modification.

Complications

• Intra-articular infection is rare—around 1 : 30 000 procedures.
• Short-term increases in pain and inflammation after injection are common, particularly with soft-tissue injection. Patients should be warned about this. This usually settles within 48 h and can be managed with analgesics. Rarely, a very florid flare in arthritis is seen, which must be differentiated from sepsis by re-aspiration.
• Tendon rupture.
• Skin atrophy and depigmentation: more common after superficial injection, with the use of potent steroids and with repeat injections.
• Facial flushing may be experienced in the hour after injection.
• Exacerbation of diabetes mellitus: changes in diabetic medication are not usually required because the effect is generally mild and transient.
• Systemic side effect of corticosteroids: adrenal suppression and iatrogenic Cushing's syndrome may occur if frequent injections are used, or if there is concurrent use of oral steroids.

 Local corticosteroid injections are generally used to minimize the systemic side effects associated with this class of drugs. However, some systemic absorption does occur and this can sometimes be therapeutically useful in the patient with a florid polyarthritis. Injection of the two to four worst affected joints will often allow sufficient systemic anti-inflammatory action to reduce more widespread joint inflammation and improve well-being, without resorting to oral steroids (which are often difficult to stop once started).

3.7 Intravenous immunoglobulin

Principle

Intravenous immunoglobulin (IVIg) therapy refers to the replacement of IgG antibodies in patients with defective B-cell function or its immunomodulatory role in autoimmune disease.

Indications

Antibody deficiency

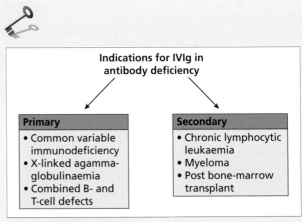

Fig. 73 Indications for IVIg in antibody deficiency.

Intravenous immunoglobulin should not be used in IgG subclass deficiency unless there is objective evidence of specific antibody deficiency and antibiotic prophylaxis has failed.

Immunomodulation

Intravenous immunoglobulin therapy has been enthusiastically tried in a wide range of diseases [1, 2], but proof of its efficacy has been demonstrated in relatively few.

 Intravenous immunoglobulin as an immunomodulatory agent

Efficacy proven in randomized controlled trials (RCT)
• Immune thrombocytopenia
• Guillain–Barré syndrome
• Chronic inflammatory demyelinating polyneuropathy
• Kawasaki's disease
• Dermatomyositis
• Lambert–Eaton syndrome

Ineffective in RCT
• Postviral fatigue (chronic fatigue syndrome)
• Rheumatoid arthritis
• Juvenile rheumatoid arthritis.

Contraindications

There are no absolute contraindications but caution should be exercised in the following:
• Patients with total IgA deficiency and anti-IgA antibodies, in view of the risk of anaphylaxis. Use an IVIg product containing low levels of IgA for such patients [3].
• Patients with pre-existing renal impairment. Infusion of high-dose IVIg may precipitate reversible renal failure in this situation.
• Untreated bacterial infection.

 Infusion of IVIg in the presence of bacterial sepsis may result in exogenous IgG complexing with bacterial antigen to cause an immune complex reaction.

Practical details

Before procedure

It is important to counsel patients on the risks and benefits of treatment with a blood product derivative. Measure hepatitis B surface antigen (HBsAg), hepatitis C RNA and save serum before the first infusion and 6 monthly. Measure liver function and trough IgG before each infusion. Ensure availability of trained assistant, injectable epinephrine and telephone if receiving home therapy.

The procedure

The usual dose is 0.4 g/kg 2–3 weekly, sufficient to keep trough IgG well within the normal range. Higher levels may be required in established bronchiectasis or if granulomatous disease is present. Infuse at 0.01–0.07 mL/kg per min. Slower rates are used when initiating treatment.

 The dose of IVIg used for immunomodulation is five times higher (2 g/kg) than that used for antibody replacement.

Observe for adverse effects. Reduce infusion rate if mild side effects occur. Discontinue if moderate or severe side effects occur.

After the procedure

Note batch number of IVIg and any adverse events.

Complications

Complications may be divided into immediate infusion-related events, those related to infusing high doses of IgG

and transmission of infections as a result of infusing a blood product [4].

Infusion-related events

Serious anaphylactoid or immune complex-mediated reactions are rare. Milder infusion-related reactions, e.g. headache, flushing, low backache, nausea, chills and abdominal pain, occur in 2–6% of cases and respond rapidly to a reduction in the rate of infusion.

Sudden rise in serum IgG

These complications are seen only with high-dose IVIg:
• Aseptic meningitis: aetiology unknown; occurs in approximately 10% of patients.
• Haemolysis caused by antiblood group antibodies: this is exceptional but may occur if IVIg contains high titres of blood group antibodies.
• Reversible renal failure as a result of osmotic tubular injury caused by the carbohydrate component of IVIg.

Blood-borne viral transmission

Stringent precautions in donor selection and plasma screening has minimized, but not eliminated, the risk of viral transmission, especially hepatitis C. Minimize risk by monitoring batch number and liver function, enabling swift recall in case of an infected batch. Do not change the IVIg preparation except for strong clinical reasons.

 HIV and hepatitis B have not been transmitted by IVIg, presumably because these viruses do not survive Cohn ethanol fractionation, the manufacturing process for IVIg.

1 Ballow M. Mechanisms of action of intravenous serum globulin in autoimmune and inflammatory diseases. *J Allergy Clin Immunol* 1997; 100: 151–157.
2 Dalakas MC. Intravenous immune globulin therapy for neurologic diseases. *Ann Intern Med* 1997; 126: 721–730.
3 Bjorkander J, Hammarström L, Edvard Smith CI *et al.* Immunoglobulin prophylaxis in patients with antibody deficiency syndromes and anti-IgA antibodies. *J Clin Immunol* 1987; 7: 8–15.
4 Misbah SA, Chapel HM. Adverse effects of intravenous immunoglobulin. *Drug Safety* 1993; 9: 254–262.

Acknowledgement

Faye Storey's sterling secretarial efforts are gratefully acknowledged.

4 Self-assessment

Answers are on pp. 121–7.

Question 1

The image (Fig. 74) shows the hand of an 18-year-old man who presents to the Accident and Emergency department with a fever and a rash. What is the probable diagnosis?

A streptococcal septicaemia

B staphylococcal septicaemia

C meningococcal septicaemia

D thrombocytopenic purpura

E acute vasculitis

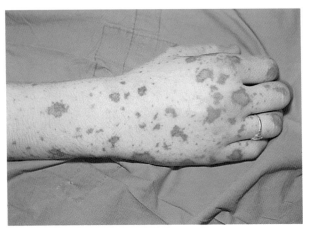

Fig. 74 Question 1. (With permission from Bannister BA, Begg NT, Gillespie SH. *Infectious Disease*, 2nd edn. Oxford: Blackwell Science, 2000.)

Question 2

Consider Table 35. A 38-year-old woman with a history of perennial rhinitis undergoes skin prick testing, which one of the following patterns of response is most likely to be hers?

A pattern 1

B pattern 2

C pattern 3

D pattern 4

E pattern 5

Question 3

An 18-year-old man is under investigation for Crohn's disease because of chronic perianal sepsis, with fistula formation after drainage of an abscess. He presents with fever. His CT scan is shown (Fig. 75). His 4-year-old brother was recently treated for a similar condition. What is the likely diagnosis?

A familial Crohn's disease

B inherited complement deficiency

C inherited neutrophil killing defect

D inherited cytokine/cytokine receptor deficiency

E inherited T-cell deficiency

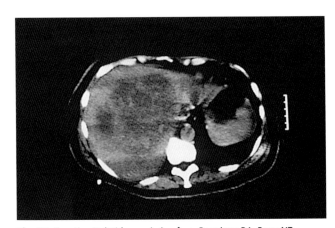

Fig. 75 Question 3. (With permission from Bannister BA, Begg NT, Gillespie SH. *Infectious Disease*, 2nd edn. Oxford: Blackwell Science, 2000.)

Question 4

A 30-year-old woman with a two-year history of Raynaud's phenomenon presents with increasing pain in her hand (Fig. 76a). Her serum is tested for antinuclear antibodies on a human epithelial cell line (HEp-2) substrate, with result shown (Fig. 76b). What is the likely diagnosis?

A Wegener's granulomatosis

B microscopic polyangiitis

C diffuse cutaneous systemic sclerosis

D limited cutaneous systemic sclerosis

E polyarteritis nodosa

	Diluent (negative) (mm)	Histamine (mm)	Grass pollen (mm)	House dust mite (mm)	Latex (mm)
1	1	7	0	4	0
2	0	4	1 + 8 of erythema	0	0
3	0	1	0	2	0
4	5	7	3	4	3
5	0	6	4	0	0

Table 35 Question 2: skinprick test results—the diameter of the weal is shown (in millimetres).

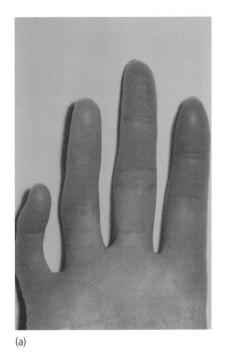
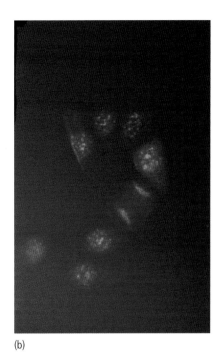

Fig. 76 Question 4.
(a)
(b)

Question 5

A 36-year-old man presents with an 8-week history of sinusitis and arthralgia. The sinusitis has not improved with prolonged antibiotic treatment. His serum CRP is markedly raised at 125 mg/l (reference range 0–10 mg/l). The appearances of his paranasal sinuses on CT scan are shown (Fig. 77a), also the results of an indirect immuno-fluorescence test of his serum using human ethanol-fixed neutrophils as a substrate (Fig. 77b). What is the likely diagnosis?

A systemic lupus erythematosus

B diffuse cutaneous systemic sclerosis

C polyarteritis nodosa

D microscopic polyangiitis

E Wegener's granulomatosis

Question 6

A 30-year-old garage mechanic presents with severe malaise that has come on over a week or so. He does not have any specific symptoms and examination is un-remarkable, excepting that he looks unwell and is pale. Blood tests confirm that he is anaemic (Hb 8.7 g/dl), also that he is in renal failure (Na 135 mmol/l, K 5.8 mmol/l, creatinine 798 µmol/l). There is patchy lung shadowing on his chest radiograph. His kidneys are of normal size on ultrasound and renal biopsy is performed to achieve a diagnosis of the cause of his renal failure. The image (Fig. 78) shows the appearance of the biopsy on immuno-fluorescent examination using an anti-IgG antibody. What is the diagnosis?

A Goodpasture's disease

B IgA nephropathy

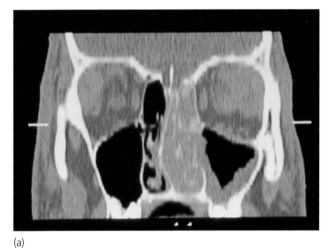

(a)

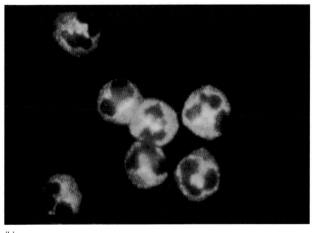

(b)

Fig. 77 Question 5.

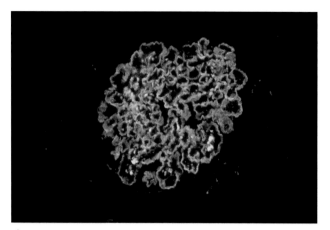

Fig. 78 Question 6.

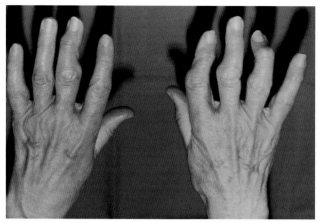

Fig. 79 Question 8.

C Wegener's granulomatosis
D membranous glomerulonephritis
E cholesterol embolisation

Question 7

A 63-year-old man with no previous history of arthritis presents with a painful, swollen knee joint. You are uncertain of the diagnosis and perform diagnostic aspiration. Which one of the fluids described in Table 36 would be compatible with the diagnosis of pseudogout, or would none of them?
A fluid A
B fluid B
C fluid C
D fluid D
E none of the fluids described

Question 8

A 58-year-old woman is referred with pain and stiffness in her hands and knees. She has a few patches of psoriasis on her arms. Her hands are shown in the picture (Fig. 79). What are the two most likely diagnoses?
A gout
B nodal osteoarthritis
C pseudogout
D systemic sclerosis
E psoriatic arthritis

F systemic lupus erythematosus
G ankylosing spondylitis
H rheumatoid arthritis
I reactive arthritis
J SAPHO syndrome

Question 9

A 30-year-old woman presents with several attacks of pain and swelling affecting the metacarpophalangeal and proximal interphalangeal joints over the past few months, with morning stiffness and fatigue. What are the two most likely diagnoses?
A ankylosing spondylitis
B pseudogout
C systemic lupus erythematosus
D primary generalised osteoarthritis
E reactive arthritis
F gout
G rheumatoid arthritis
H psoriatic arthropathy
I systemic sclerosis
J rheumatic fever

Question 10

A 75-year-old woman presents with a 24-hour history of a painful swollen right knee. She feels generally unwell and has a temperature of 38.1°C. She has had minor pain and

Table 36 Question 7: synovial fluid analyses.

	Fluid A	Fluid B	Fluid C	Fluid D
Macroscopic appearance	Clear	Turbid	Turbid	Turbid
Microscopy	<1000 cells/mm^3	50 000 cells/mm^3, mainly neutrophils	60 000 cells/mm^3, mainly neutrophils	125 000 cells/mm^3, mainly neutrophils
	No crystals	Needle-shaped crystals	No crystals	Large numbers
Culture	No organisms Sterile	No organisms Sterile	No organisms Sterile	Gram-positive cocci *Staphylococcus aureus* +++

stiffness in both knees for many years. Select the most likely diagnosis, and the diagnosis that requires rapid exclusion.

A gout
B rheumatoid arthritis
C primary generalised osteoarthritis
D pseudogout
E reactive arthritis
F osteonecrosis
G haemarthrosis
H avascular necrosis
I septic arthritis
J haemochromatosis

Question 11

A 34-year-old man presents with severe low back pain, which has forced him to stop work as a bus driver. He has had back pain on and off for many years, on occasion with right-sided sciatica. The pain used to be helped by rest, but is now present more or less all the time and is stopping him from sleeping properly. The most likely diagnosis is:

A mechanical back pain
B ankylosing spondylitis
C myeloma
D osteoporosis
E osteoarthritis

Question 12

A 73-year-old man presents with a 24-hour history of a painful swollen left knee. He has had minor pain and stiffness in both knees for many years and now feels generally unwell. His temperature is 37.4°C. The most likely diagnosis is:

A gout
B pseudogout
C septic arthritis
D reactive arthritis
E rheumatoid arthritis

Question 13

A 60-year-old woman develops acute, severe low thoracic back pain. A radiograph shows a vertebral crush fracture. Which two of the following reduce an individual's risk for developing osteoporosis?

A early menarche
B early menopause
C smoking
D high alcohol intake
E prolonged treatment with corticosteroids
F rheumatoid arthritis
G Crohn's disease
H asthma
I frequent walks
J obesity

Question 14

A 20-year-old man with common variable antibody deficiency presents to the Accident and Emergency department with a 3-day history of cough productive of green sputum. His temperature is 37.5°C, pulse 84/min, respiratory rate 12/min, and breath sounds are vesicular. The chest radiograph is unremarkable. Which two immediate actions do you recommend?

A prescribe a 14-day course of antibiotics
B prescribe nebulised salbutamol
C give an infusion of intravenous immunoglobulin
D take a sputum sample to look for acid fast bacilli
E prescribe a 5-day course of antibiotics
F check his serum immunoglobulin levels
G choose an antibiotic regimen suitable for possible pseudomonas infection
H order a high resolution CT scan
I take a sputum sample for culture
J prescribe a 28-day course of antibiotics

Question 15

A 48-year-old woman with a 10-year history of systemic sclerosis presents with exertional breathlessness. Serial peak flow rates are normal. A plain chest radiograph is reported as normal and pulmonary function tests reveal reduced gas transfer with a KCO 50% of predicted. Her haemoglobin is normal. She has never smoked. Which two of the following investigations are most likely to be helpful in determining the cause of her breathlessness?

A antinuclear antibody
B high resolution CT scan of the thorax
C antibodies to extractable nuclear antigens
D 24-hour blood pressure monitoring
E V/Q scanning
F serum lactate
G muscle biopsy
H barium swallow
I trial of corticosteroid treatment
J diaphragmatic function tests

Question 16

A 27-year-old woman has a 6-year history of systemic lupus erythematosus (SLE) treated with azathioprine, hydroxychloroquine and prednisolone. She presents with a 2-week history of slowly worsening severe pain and restriction of the right hip. Which two of the following diagnoses seem most likely?

A gout
B flare of systemic lupus erythematosus (SLE)
C secondary osteoarthritis
D Perthe's disease
E septic arthritis
F secondary fibromyalgia
G irritable hip

H osteoporotic fracture of femoral neck

I avascular necrosis of the femoral head

J slipped upper femoral epiphysis

Question 17

A 79-year-old man presents feeling very unwell with recent and sudden onset of severe pain and stiffness around his shoulders and hips. He was previously well and admits to no other symptoms, in particular no headache or visual disturbance. Examination shows painful, restricted shoulders and hips, but no myopathy. He has no lymph nodes or abdominal masses. Initial investigations show a normal blood count, biochemical profile, thyroid function, prostate specific antigen, MSU and chest radiograph. His ESR is 85 mm and CRP is 110 mg/l (normal < 10). Which two of the following statements give the best advice regarding his treatment? He should:

A be started on prednisolone 60 mg daily reduced over 12–18 months

B be treated with a Cox II inhibitor

C be started on prednisolone 15 mg daily for 2 weeks only

D be treated with alfacalcidol 2 µg daily

E be treated with low dose methotrexate

F be started on prednisolone 15 mg daily, tailed off over 12–18 months

G receive 3×1 g doses of i.v. methylprednisolone

H receive prophylactic treatment for osteoporosis

I receive simple analgesia

J receive prednisolone 60 mg daily for 1 month

Question 18

You are called to the Accident and Emergency department to review a 28-year-old woman with pleuritic chest pain. Which one of the following statements concerning this patient is true?

A low white cell count is consistent with systemic lupus erythematosus (SLE)

B low white cell count is not consistent with tuberculosis.

C the presence of anticardiolipin antibodies IgG 17 GPLU/ml (NR < 14), IgM 21 MPLU/ml (NR < 10) suggests that she may have a pulmonary embolus

D the presence of antinuclear antibodies at a titre of 1/80 suggests that she may have a connective tissue disease

E the presence of antinuclear cytoplasmic antibodies (cANCA) at a titre of 1 in 20 suggests that Wegener's granulomatosis is likely

Question 19

The parents of a 10-year-old asthmatic boy with peanut allergy are concerned about the risk of future anaphylaxis if he were to inadvertently ingest peanuts. Which of the following features is the single most important predictor of anaphylaxis in this situation?

A level of peanut-specific IgE in his serum

B strength of positive skin test response to peanut

C poorly controlled asthma

D previous steroid therapy

E family history of nut allergy

Question 20

A 34-year-old woman presents to your clinic complaining of cold hands, particularly in the winter months. On examination she has cold dusky hands and a petechial rash. Investigations are as follows: Hb 10.9 g/dL; WBC 4.2×10^9/L; platelets 407×10^9/L; urea and electrolytes—normal; liver function tests—normal; albumin 36 g/L; globulin 90 g/L; Protein electrophoresis—polyclonal increase in gammaglobulins; antinuclear antibodies present (1/160, speckled pattern); complement—C3 0.79 (NR 0.75–1.25), C4 < 0.04 (NR 0.14–0.6). Which one of the following statements is true?

A active systemic lupus erythematous (SLE) is unlikely if DNA antibodies are present

B a blood sample sent to the lab on ice may show cryoglobulins

C Sjögren's syndrome is unlikely if rheumatoid factor is present

D Sjögren's syndrome is likely if Ro and La extractable nuclear antigens are present

E hepatitis C is unlikely in this case

Question 21

A 28-year-old man has recently been discharged from hospital after treatment for pneumococcal pneumonia. He has had repeated courses of antibiotics for sinus, ear and lower respiratory tract infections, and had sinus surgery the previous year. He is a life-long non-smoker and is not on medication. His blood count prior to discharge was normal. In the absence of further clues in the history or examination, which single blood test is the most important?

A HIV antibody test

B pneumococcal antibodies

C immunoglobulin levels

D liver function tests

E IgG subclass levels

Question 22

A 20-year-old woman presents with sudden onset of swelling of the lips and tongue. She also has attacks of abdominal pain and vomiting, which her mother confirms have occurred intermittently over many years. A brother and older sister have the same disorder. Which one of the following statements about this disease is accurate?

A it has sex-linked inheritance

B animal allergen is often identified in the house

C serum C4 levels are often low

D antinuclear antibodies (ANA) is often positive

E raised IgE helps differentiate it from other immune disorders

Question 23

A 60-year-old accountant complains of recurrent attacks of exquisite pain and swelling in the left big toe. Which of the following conditions is NOT likely to be associated with this disorder?

A chronic alcoholism

B obesity

C rheumatoid arthritis

D diabetes mellitus

E diuretic therapy

Question 24

A 20-year-old man presents with arthralgia, skin rash and haematuria. Renal biopsy shows focal necrotising glomerulonephritis with diffuse mesangial IgA deposits. What is the most likely diagnosis?

A systemic lupus erythematosus (SLE)

B Henoch–Schönlein purpura

C juvenile rheumatoid arthritis

D post-streptococcal glomerulonephritis

E Goodpasture's syndrome

Question 25

A 65-year-old woman with a mitral valve replacement presents to the Accident and Emergency department with pyrexia and fainting. She is unwell, hypotensive, anaemic and pyrexial. She has a vague history of suffering from a reaction to penicillin in her childhood. After taking blood cultures she is started on broad-spectrum antibiotics. Cardiac valvular vegetations are seen on echocardiography and her blood grows methicillin-sensitive *Staphylococci*. The microbiologist suggests naficillin as the most appropriate antibiotic, but is concerned that she may have an allergy to beta lactam-based antibiotics. Which of the following is most appropriate to investigate the history of possible penicillin allergy?

A serum tryptase

B skin prick test to penicillin

C serum penicillin specific IgE

D patch test to penicillin

E serum IgE

Question 26

A 36-year-old woman is referred with a 1-year history of muscle pain, tiredness and sleep disturbance. She denies fever, weight loss and arthralgia. Examination reveals tenderness over her occiput, trapezius and lumbar area. Her blood results show a normal ESR, CRP, FBC, a weakly positive ANA (1:80) and normal complement levels. What is the most likely diagnosis?

A polymyositis

B system lupus erythematous (SLE)

C Sjögren's syndrome

D polymyalgia rheumatica

E fibromyalgia

Question 27

A 30-year-old female nurse presents with a 3-month history of Raynaud's phenomenon. Clinical examination reveals cold hands but no other evidence of connective tissue disease. Which of the following tests is most helpful in determining future progression to systemic connective tissue disease?

A positive anti-mitochondrial antibody

B positive anti-gastric parietal cell antibody

C positive smooth muscle antibody

D positive anti-nuclear antibody

E positive rheumatoid factor

Question 28

A 30-year-old woman presents with a 6-month history of swelling and pain involving the distal interphalangeal joints of the hands. The ESR is 65 mm in the first hour. What is the most likely diagnosis?

A generalised osteoarthritis

B rheumatoid arthritis

C psoriatic arthritis

D systemic lupus erythematosus (SLE)

E gout

Question 29

A 28-year-old woman presents with fatigue and extreme tiredness. Physical examination reveals facial skin rash and tenderness across the small joints of the hands. She is concerned that she might have systemic lupus erythematosus (SLE). Which one of the following tests will virtually exclude the diagnosis of SLE as cause for her symptoms if it is NEGATIVE?

A antinuclear antibody (ANA)

B anti-double stranded DNA

C anti-Sm antibodies

D anti-histone antibodies

E anti-Ro/SS-A antibodies

Question 30

A 66-year-old woman has a 15-year history of deforming rheumatoid arthritis (RA) for which she takes D-penicillamine. Two weeks ago she noticed increased difficulty in climbing stairs and three days before admission she was unable to comb her hair or feed herself. Neurological assessment reveals weakness in arms and legs. Both plantars are upgoing. Which one of the following tests is most likely to provide the diagnosis?

A plain radiograph of the cervical spine

B electromyography (EMG)

C nerve conduction study (NCS)

D isotope bone scan

E magnetic resonance imaging (MRI) of the cervical spine

Question 31

A 68-year old man presents with sudden severe pain and swelling in the left knee. Synovial fluid analysis shows abundant calcium pyrophosphate dihydrate (CPPD) crystals. In his further assessment, which one of the following tests is NOT appropriate?

A creatinine kinase

B serum calcium

C thyroid function test

D serum ferritin level

E HbA$_1$C

Question 32

A 35-year-old man is referred for investigation of recurrent infection. He has had frequent respiratory tract infections for the past 5 years, requiring 4–5 courses of antibiotics each winter. A month previously he was admitted with pneumococcal pneumonia, and two months prior to that he had sinus surgery. Which of the following conditions is NOT in the differential diagnosis?

A antibody deficiency

B HIV infection

C bronchiectasis secondary to recurrent infection

D complement C6 deficiency

E smoking 5 cigarettes per day

Question 33

A 19-year-old woman presents with fever and cough. Sputum samples are negative on microscopy for acid fast bacilli, but six weeks later *M. tuberculosis* (MTB) is grown. She completed a course of chemotherapy for pulmonary TB two months previously. Her chest radiograph is unchanged from one taken at this time. Which of the following is the most likely explanation for these findings?

A she has HIV co-infection causing increased susceptibility to mycobacteria

B the organism isolated is a contaminant

C she has been re-infected with a different strain of TB

D she has underlying IFNγ receptor deficiency causing increased susceptibility to mycobacteria.

E she has been poorly adherent to therapy and her TB has recurred

Question 34

A 68-year-old woman with longstanding congestive cardiac failure (ejection fraction 20%) presents with a hot, swollen right knee. The following results are obtained: FBC normal, Urea 11 mM, Creatinine 196 μmol/l. Synovial fluid: many monosodium urate crystals seen on microscopy, culture sterile. What is the best treatment for her acute arthritis?

A allopurinol

B colchicine 0.5 mg every 2–4 hours

C indometacin 50 mg tds

D co-codamol 30/500 every 6 hours

E intra-articular corticosteroids

Question 35

A 65-year-old woman presents with a 3-month history of recurrent attacks of facial angioedema. Which of the following test results would favour a diagnosis of C1 inhibitor deficiency?

A low complement C3 levels and a normal C4

B low complement C4 levels and a normal C3

C hypergammaglobulinaemia

D hypogammaglobulinaemia

E positive rheumatoid factor

Question 36

A 30-year-old woman develops a systemic reaction characterised by hypotension, bronchospasm and widespread urticaria soon after induction of anaesthesia for cholecystectomy. Which of the following blood test results would suggest that her reaction was associated with mast cell degranulation?

A elevated plasma tryptase

B hypernatraemia

C hypokalaemia

D hypocomplementaemia

E hypergammaglobulinaemia

Question 37

A 70-year-old woman has a 17-year history of rheumatoid arthritis. She presents with recurrent attacks of red congested eyes with a sensation of grittiness. The most likely cause of her red eyes is likely to be:

A scleritis

B episcleritis

C keratitis

D keratoconjunctivitis sicca

E choroiditis

Question 38

A 77-year-old man presents with persistent headache and progressive deafness. On examination he has frontal bossing of the forehead and conductive deafness, more severe in the right ear. His serum alkaline phosphatase is significantly raised at 870 Iu/L. Which of the following statements is most accurate about this disease?

A it usually affects a single bone

B the skull is the most commonly affected bone

C bone pain is the most common presenting feature

D hearing loss is often due to involvement of the middle ear ossicles leading to conductive deafness
E bone pain is typically increased with rest and on weight bearing

Question 39

A 50-year-old man gives an 8-month history of episodic, painful soft tissue swellings involving his hands, eyes and lips. There is no temporal relationship to food. Which of the following tests is the most useful?
A skin prick tests to various food allergens
B Serum complement
C full blood count (FBC)
D glucose tolerance test
E urinary 5-hydroxyindoleacetic acid

Question 40

A 64-year-old man presents to the Accident and Emergency department with a 2-day history of increasing pain and swelling of his left knee. He denies a history of trauma. On examination, the knee is hot, red, swollen and extremely tender. Which of the following investigations is most important?
A plain radiograph of the knee
B blood cultures
C C-reactive protein (CRP)
D joint aspiration
E plasma uric acid level

Answers to Self-assessment

Answer to Question 1

C

With this history, the diagnosis is meningococcal septicaemia. This is a fulminant disease, delay of a few hours can be fatal, and immediate treatment with intravenous benzylpenicillin or cefotaxime should be given.

Meningococcal septicaemia can affect a normal host, but patients with a deficiency of a terminal complement component are particularly susceptible. This can most easily be detected by measuring the CH50 or CH100, which tests the ability of the complement in the patient's serum to lyse erythrocytes by the classical complement pathway. If any complement component (C1-9) is missing, lysis will not occur.

Answer to Question 2

A

Pattern 1 is that of a patient with perennial rhinitis, which is commonly due to house dust mite allergy; pattern 2 is normal; pattern 3 would be typical of a patient taking antihistamines; pattern 4 of someone with dermatographism; pattern 5 is of a patient with hayfever due to grass pollen allergy.

Oral histamines should be discontinued for 4 days (4 weeks in the case of astemizole) before skin prick testing because, as shown, they can mask reactions. Areas of induration more than 3 mm in diameter greater than that of the negative control are considered to be positive: the area of erythema is not measured.

Answer to Question 3

C

The CT shows a large multilocular liver abscess. This, together with the family history and the perianal abscess, suggest an inherited neutrophil killing defect, such as chronic granulomatous disease.

The nitroblue tetrazolium (NBT) test is used as a screening test for neutrophil killing defects, when the neutrophils fail to reduce NBT that they have phagocytosed, which remains in the neutrophils as dark blue crystals.

Answer to Question 4

D

The hand is critically ischaemic with impending gangrene. The pattern of immunofluorescence is typical of an anticentromere antibody, with multiple fine dots due to staining of the kinetochores of the 23 pairs of chromosomes. In this clinical context, anticentromere antibodies are reliable markers of the CREST syndrome (Calcinosis, Raynaud's, Esophageal dysfunction, Sclerodactyly, Telangiectasia), also known as limited cutaneous systemic sclerosis.

Answer to Question 5

E

The CT scan shows soft tissue masses occupying the left nasal cavity, left ethmoid sinus, left maxillary antrum, and both orbits. The staining of neutrophils shows granular fluorescence of the cytoplasm typical of c-ANCA that in this clinical context virtually clinches the diagnosis of Wegener's granulomatosis, which would be confirmed by a specific test for antibodies directed against proteinase-3 (PR3-ANCA).

Answer to Question 6

A

The kidney biopsy shows striking linear deposits of IgG along the glomerular basement membrane (GBM), indicating the presence of anti-GBM antibodies diagnostic (in this clinical context) of Goodpasture's disease.

Answer to Question 7

E

Fluid A would be typical of osteoarthritis; fluid B of gout; fluid C of a non-crystal associated inflammatory arthritis (e.g. rheumatoid, reactive, psoriatic); fluid D of septic arthritis. The crystals in the joint in pseudogout are made of calcium pyrophosphate, which are rhomboid or rectangular and not needle shaped.

Answer to Question 8

B, E

Swelling of the distal interphalangeal joints really only occurs in nodal osteoarthritis and one of the forms of psoriatic arthritis, which is usually easily distinguished by nail involvement (not present in this case).

Involvement of the base of the thumb is also pathognomonic of nodal osteoarthritis, giving the thumb base a characteristically square appearance.

Answer to Question 9

C, G

The most likely cause of these symptoms is rheumatoid arthritis, but SLE requires careful consideration.

Rheumatoid arthritis can present as an acute monoarthritis, an acute polyarthritis, a subacute insidious polyarthritis, or with a polymyalgic presentation (particularly in the elderly, when it needs to be differentiated from polymyalgia rheumatica).

Remember that acute synovitis in early rheumatoid arthritis is associated with very little fixed joint deformity and no extra-articular features. This contrasts with the deforming arthritis that is characteristic of chronic disease.

Answer to Question 10

D, I

The primary concern in the assessment of the acute hot

joint is to exclude septic arthritis, hence diagnostic aspiration of synovial fluid is the essential urgent investigation. Grossly purulent fluid suggests sepsis; blood-stained fluid may indicate haemarthrosis but can also occur in pseudogout, which is the likeliest cause of this presentation.

An acute hot joint in an elderly person is most often due to crystal arthritis, whereas a reactive arthritis is more probable in a sexually active young adult.

Answer to Question 11

A

The history is typical of a patient with mechanical back pain, best treated by encouraging mobilisation, simple analgaesia, a graded rehabilitative exercise programme and treatment of depression (if present).

'Red flag' symptoms, requiring urgent investigation to exclude sinister pathology, include: age >55 or <18 yr, progressive pain, night pain, systemic symptoms, progressive neurological deficit, past history of malignancy or immunosuppression, and recent trauma.

Answer to Question 12

B

It would be important to exclude septic arthritis by microscopy and culture of fluid aspirated from the knee, but this is not the commonest cause of an acute monoarthritis.

The differential diagnosis is influenced by age. Crystal arthritis is the most common cause in elderly people, whereas reactive arthritis tends to occur in sexually active young adults.

Calcium pyrophosphate deposition disease, often known as pseudogout, can often present with striking fever and systemic illness. Treatment is with NSAIDs or intra-articular steroid injection, once sepsis has been excluded.

Answer to Question 13

A, I

The most likely cause of a vertebral crush factor in a woman of this age is obviously osteoporosis, but local vertebral pathology—in particular secondary tumours or myeloma—would need to be considered.

It is most likely that the cause of osteoporosis would be 'postmenopausal' in this woman, but many medical factors influence the likelihood of this condition.

The following tests should be considered in a patient presenting with an osteoporotic fracture (although not all need to be performed in all cases): full blood count, renal/liver/bone chemistry, immunoglobulins and serum/urine electrophoresis (to exclude myeloma), thyroid function, testosterone (in men), investigations for Cushing's syndrome.

Answer to Question 14

A, I

Antibody deficient patients need prompt treatment of presumed bacterial infection. Treatment should be continued for longer than normal: 14 days for an uncomplicated chest infection would be appropriate. Most infections are caused by common organisms such as haemophilus or pneumococcus: psuedomonas is unusual and mycobacterial disease rare in common variable immunodeficiency. Cultures are invaluable if there is a poor response to treatment and for guiding future antibiotic choices. For infections causing fever, routine antibody replacement should be deferred for 24–48 hours until there is a clear response to treatment, as adverse reactions are much more common in the presence of fever.

Answer to Question 15

B, E

The important complications of systemic sclerosis to consider are interstitial lung disease, pulmonary hypertension and cardiac disease (usually myocardial, sometimes pericardial). Pulmonary emboli are fairly common in the context of connective tissue disease, especially when cardiolipin antibodies are present. Diaphragmatic weakness can occur, due to myopathy, but would not produce marked reduction in gas transfer.

Answer to Question 16

E, I

The most likely diagnosis is avascular necrosis, the risk factors for this being corticosteroids and SLE itself, particularly in patients with anti-cardiolipin antibodies. Sepsis is less likely but possible: it must be excluded. The risk of sepsis is increased by immunosuppression, which may also modify the presentation—less fever, more insidious onset, and bloods may be normal.

This patient is at increased risk of osteoporosis but a hip fracture would be a very rare event at this age, and would usually be associated with sudden onset of pain rather than insidious onset. Osteoarthritis due to synovitis is almost never seen in SLE which produces a non-erosive arthritis.

Answer to Question 17

F, H

The diagnosis is polymyalgia rheumatica. This will usually respond dramatically to small doses of prednisolone, which will be required for an average duration of 12–18 months before the disease goes into remission. The major side effect of such low doses of steroid is osteoporosis and prophylaxis will usually be required.

Answer to Question 18
A

Active SLE and tuberculosis are both associated with leukopenia. Low titre antinuclear antibodies (in the absence of DNA or ENA), antineutrophil cytoplasmic antibodies (ANCA) and anticardiolipin antibodies are non-specific and are commonly found in the presence of infection.

Answer to Question 19
C

Poorly controlled asthma is an important risk factor for fatal anaphylaxis in this situation and all efforts necessary should be made to ensure that asthma is well controlled. Parents and children (when old enough) should be taught how to recognise the early symptoms and signs of anaphylaxis, how to administer self-injectable adrenaline, and should always have this available.

Answer to Question 20
D

The symptoms, signs and low C4 are suggestive of cryoglobulinaemia. Sludging of proteins at reduced temperatures – as might occur in the hands on a cold day—can cause ischaemia and sometimes vasculitis. Cryoglobulinaemia is commonly associated with hepatitis C or connective tissue disease, such as Sjögren's syndrome. The positive ANA and high globulins suggest Sjögren's in this case, but could also be associated with chronic infection, such as hepatitis C.

Since they precipitate at low temperatures, cryoglobulins should always be transported to the lab at 37°C. Failure to do this will result in a false negative result as the cryos will precipitate and be removed with the clot.

Answer to Question 21
C

Hypogammaglobulinaemia is associated with recurrent bacterial infections, most commonly of the respiratory tract. Delay of several years prior to diagnosis is usual, with associated morbidity. Patients with low immunoglobulin levels and recurrent infections should be treated with immunoglobulin replacement. More minor antibody defects, such as IgG subclass or specific antibody (to pneumococcus) defects can often be treated with appropriate vaccinations and/or prophylactic antibiotics.

Answer to Question 22
C

Hereditary angioneurotic oedema is an autosomal dominant condition caused by a deficiency of C1 esterase inhibitor, resulting in intermittent episodes of spontaneous complement activation. Clinically the patient suffers oedema of the skin and mucosal surfaces. Fatalities may occur if the airway is compromised. C4 levels are typically low during an attack but may be normal in between attacks.

Acquired angioedema is associated with allergic reactions, often associated with urticaria, and very commonly (94% of cases) drug-induced, most frequently by angiotensin-converting enzyme (ACE) inhibitors. Insect stings and foods are other predisposing factors.

Answer to Question 23
C

Acute gout is intensely inflammatory and causes severe pain, redness, swelling and disability. At least 80% of initial attacks involve a single joint, typically in the leg or foot, most often the base of the great toe (first metatarsophalangeal joint, known as podagra) or the knee. Trauma, surgery, starvation, alcohol, dietary overindulgence and ingestion of drugs, most commonly diuretics (also cyclosporin and low dose aspirin), may all promote gouty attacks. Diabetes mellitus, obesity, hyperparathyroidism and hypothyroidism are associated with gout, but rheumatoid arthritis is not associated with hyperuricaemia or gout.

Answer to Question 24
B

Henoch–Schönlein purpura (HSP) is characterised by the tissue deposition of IgA-containing immune complexes. The pathogenesis of this disorder appears similar to that of IgA nephropathy, which is associated with identical histologic findings in the kidney.

HSP is commoner in children than in adults. Many cases follow an upper respiratory tract infection, suggesting that the precipitating antigen may be infectious. The clinical manifestations include a classic tetrad of rash, arthralgias, abdominal pain, and renal disease that can occur in any order and at any time over a period of several days to several weeks. The rash is typically purpuric and distributed symmetrically over the lower legs and arms: clotting studies are normal.

Answer to Question 25
B

A history of penicillin allergy is relatively common. In most cases it is not due to a type I hypersensitivity reaction. Diagnosis of penicillin allergy crucially requires a detailed history of the drug reaction and can be confirmed by a positive skin prick test to the major and minor determinants of penicillin. Skin prick testing is carried out if there is a clinical need for penicillin treatment e.g. treatment of infective endocarditis. A patient is unlikely to develop anaphylaxis with a negative penicillin skin prick test. The detection of penicillin specific IgE in the serum is unreliable.

Answer to Question 26

E

The lack of constitutional symptoms, normal inflammatory markers and normal examination, apart from evidence of tender points, make an inflammatory rheumatological disease unlikely. The presence of tender points, history of muscle pain and sleep disturbance are suggestive of fibromyalgia—a non-inflammatory pain disorder.

Answer to Question 27

D

Although 5% of the general population have Raynaud's phenomenon, only a minority go on to develop systemic connective tissue disease. A positive ANA is the single best predictor of existing or future progression to connective tissue disease in this situation.

Answer to Question 28

C

Arthritis with predominant involvement of the distal interphalangeal joint occurs most often in generalised osteoarthritis and psoriatic arthritis. The fact that this patient is relatively young and has a raised ESR indicates an underlying inflammatory disease is the most likely cause of her symptoms, hence psoriatic arthritis is the most likely diagnosis in this case. Examination of the skin and nails for psoriasis is very important in confirming the diagnosis. The scalp hairline, the naval and the palms are areas often involved in psoriasis but easily missed.

Rheumatoid arthritis and SLE are known to affect the proximal interphalangeal (PIPs) and the metacarpophalangeal (MCPs) joints. Chronic gouty arthritis might involve the DIPs, but more often it involves the MCPs and PIPs in asymmetrical fashion with or without tophus formation.

Answer to Question 29

A

Almost all patients with SLE have a positive ANA, which is a sensitive for SLE, but not specific. A negative result argues strongly against a diagnosis of active SLE, but does not exclude the possibility of other autoimmune diseases.

Antibodies to Sm antigen are highly specific for a diagnosis of SLE (>99%), but only about 25% of patients with SLE have anti-Sm antibodies. Anti-DNA antibodies are diagnostic of SLE (specificity > 99%), but only 60% of patients with SLE will have these antibodies. Absence of anti-DNA or anti-Sm antibodies cannot exclude SLE as a diagnosis. Anti-Ro/SS-A antibodies are found in 30% of patients with SLE. Anti-histone antibodies are identified in few SLE patients, most often those with drug-induced lupus.

Answer to Question 30

E

The recent limb weakness with pyramidal signs (upgoing plantars) in the legs in a patient with RA is very suggestive of spinal cord compression, most likely in the neck since RA primarily affects the cervical spine. The anatomic abnormalities occur as a consequence of the destruction of synovial joints, ligaments and bone, with atlantoaxial subluxation most common. Patients may experience generalised weakness, difficulty walking, paresthesias of the hands, and loss of fine dexterity. Many neurological signs may be elicited, including diffuse hyperreflexia, spasticity of the legs, a spastic gait and Babinski's sign.

Answer to Question 31

A

Pseudogout occurs when there are acute attacks of CPPD crystal-induced synovitis, which clinically resembles acute gout caused by urate crystals. However, most patients with CPPD crystal deposition in their joints never experience such episodes. A variety of metabolic and endocrine disorders are associated with CPPD crystal deposition, including diabetes mellitus, haemochromatosis, Wilson's disease, hypothyroidism, hyperparathyroidism, hypomagnesaemia and hypophosphatasia.

Answer to Question 32

D

Antibody deficiency is typically associated with respiratory tract infections. Ask about diarrhoea and bacterial skin infections which are also common. Take a careful drug history and bear in mind the possibility of lymphoproliferative disease.

HIV infection, although primarily associated with CD4 loss, also results in antibody dysfunction leading to recurrent respiratory tract infections in some patients. Ask about features of cellular immune deficiency (oral candida, herpes simplex and zoster, warts), also about risk factors.

Recurrent bacterial chest infections, whatever their cause, will eventually result in bronchiectasis, hence the importance of early diagnosis and treatment.

Terminal complement deficiencies (C5-9) are extremely rare. Patients are well but have increased susceptibility to neisserial infection.

Smoking causes ciliary paralysis, with the resultant mucociliary dysfunction a common (and reversible) cause of recurrent respiratory tract infection.

Answer to Question 33

E

Poor adherence is a common cause of treatment failure or early relapse: directly observed therapy (DOT) may improve adherence if this is the case.

TB usually responds well to conventional treatment even if the patient is co-infected with HIV. In this situation, recurrent TB is most often caused by poor adherence (early) or reinfection (late).

Underlying IFNγ receptor/ IL12 deficiency is extremely rare and is associated with disseminated disease, usually with poorly pathogenic environmental mycobacteria. Environmental mycobacteria may occasionally grow as contaminants in culture, but it is most unusual for MTB to do so.

Answer to Question 34

E

This patient has acute gout, probably diuretic-induced. Intra-articular corticosteroids are safe and highly efficacious in this situation, once sepsis is excluded.

Allopurinol has no role in the acute treatment of gout. Colchicine at these doses is very poorly tolerated due to GI toxicity. Non-steroidals are very likely to precipitate deterioration in renal function and may also exacerbate heart failure.

Answer to Question 35

B

The hallmark of all forms of C1 inhibitor deficiency is a reduced C4 with normal C3, which is a consequence of uncontrolled activation of the complement classical pathway. At this age the most likely diagnosis is acquired C1 inhibitor deficiency associated with lymphoproliferative disease or more rarely autoantibodies to C1 inhibitor.

Answer to Question 36

A

The constellation of acute symptoms is typical of a systemic allergic reaction, either anaphylaxis (if IgE mediated) or an anaphylactoid reaction (if non-IgE mediated). Both of these reactions are due to extensive mast cell degranulation leading to release of large amounts of tryptase into the circulation. Elevated tryptase levels in this clinical context are very suggestive of an anaphylactic/ anaphylactoid reaction.

This woman will need to be investigated during convalescence in an allergy clinic to determine the cause of her reaction.

Answer to Question 37

D

About 25% of patients with rheumatoid arthritis (RA)

have ocular manifestations, including keratoconjunctivitis sicca, scleritis, episcleritis, keratitis, peripheral corneal ulceration and other less common entities such as choroiditis, retinal vasculitis, episcleral nodules, retinal detachments and macular oedema.

Keratoconjunctivitis sicca, or dry eye syndrome, presents as 'gritty eyes' and is the most common ocular manifestation of RA (prevalence 15–25 %).

Answer to Question 38

E

Paget's disease is a focal disorder of bone remodelling characterised by an increase in the number and size of osteoclasts in affected skeletal sites, whilst the rest of the skeleton is spared. It can affect any bone, but the axial skeleton, particularly the pelvis, is usual. In most cases at least two bones are affected. Hearing loss through compression of the 8th nerve occurs in 30–40% of patients. Other causes of hearing loss include pagetic involvement of the middle ear ossicles, but this is relatively rare.

Unlike osteoarthritis, pagetic bone pain usually increases with rest, on weight bearing, when the limbs are warmed, and at night, but 70% or so of patients with Paget's disease have no symptoms, the diagnosis being found incidentally by radiographs and laboratory investigations.

Answer to Question 39

B

The most likely diagnosis in this patient is chronic idiopathic angioedema. However, the rarer C1-inhibitor deficiency has to be considered and would be excluded by a normal C4 level. The lack of any temporal relationship of his symptoms to the ingestion of any food excludes an allergic cause, which only rarely presents as chronic angioedema.

Answer to Question 40

D

Aspiration of the knee with microscopy to look for pus cells / organisms in the case of septic arthritis and crystals in the case of gout or pseudogout is the most useful investigation. Blood cultures may yield an organism. A radiograph would be useful as a baseline but is unlikely to show acute changes and is not the top priority. Uric acid levels may not be elevated in an acute episode of gout. A raised CRP is non-specific, but can be used to monitor the effectiveness of treatment.

The Medical Masterclass series

Clinical Skills

General Clinical Issues

Pain Relief and Palliative Care

Medicine for the Elderly

Emergency Medicine

Infectious Diseases and Dermatology

Infectious Diseases

Cardiology and Respiratory Medicine

Cardiology

Respiratory Medicine

Gastroenterology and Hepatology

Neurology, Ophthalmology and Psychiatry

Neurology

Nephrology

Rheumatology and Clinical Immunology

Index